MAD ABOUT RAW

EXCLUSIVELY DESIGNED RAW FOOD RECIPES

PHOTOGRAPHY
by NAZLI DEVELI

DESIGN
by STUDIO AURORA

EDITOR
STELLA NILSSON

First published in June 2021

Hardcover Edition - Expanded Second Printing, February 2022
ISBN 9781736374283
Independently published by Nazlı Develi

www.gurmevegan.com
www.greenandawake.com

MAD ABOUT RAW

EXCLUSIVELY DESIGNED RAW FOOD RECIPES

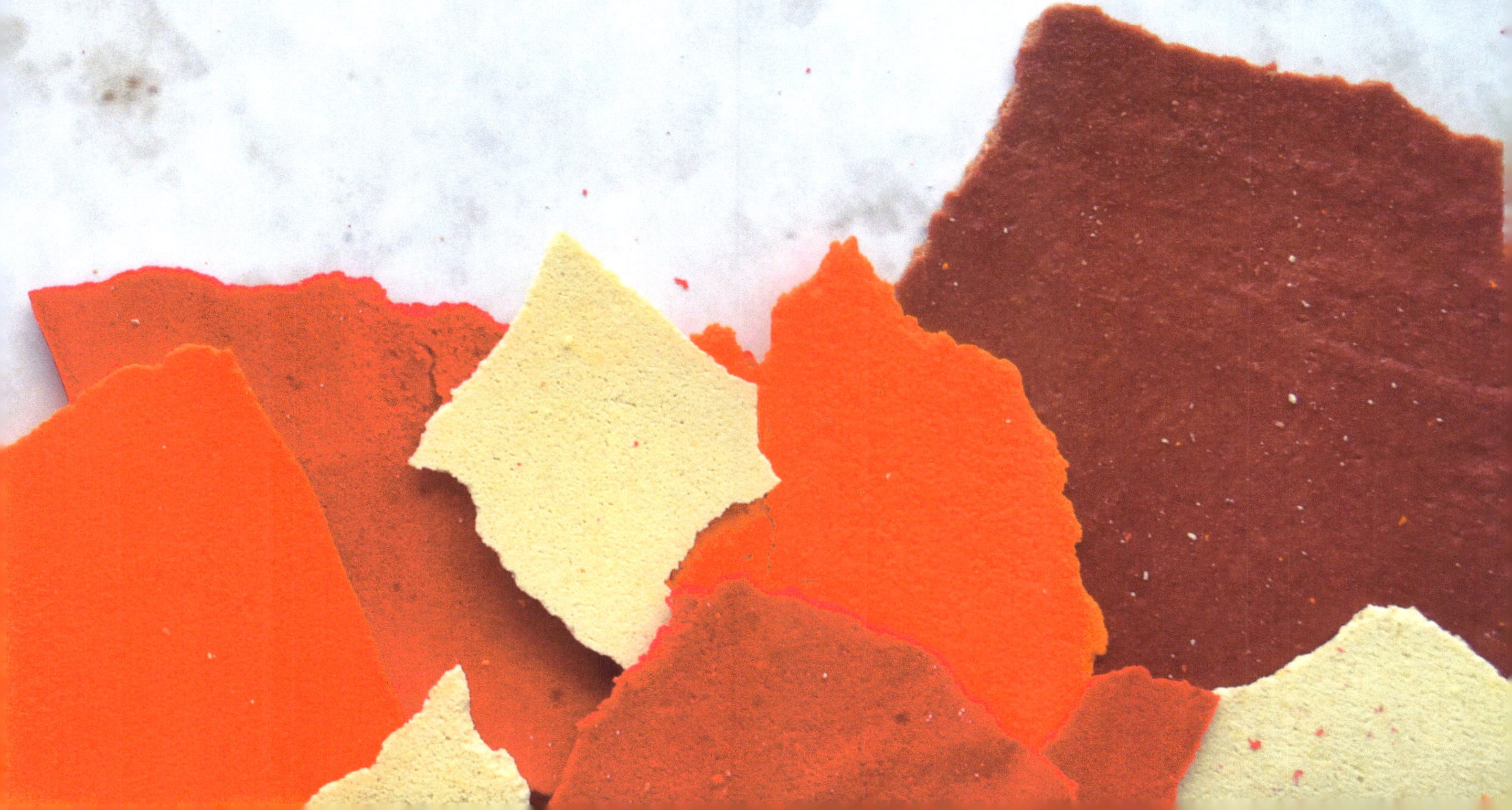

golden latte and biscotti

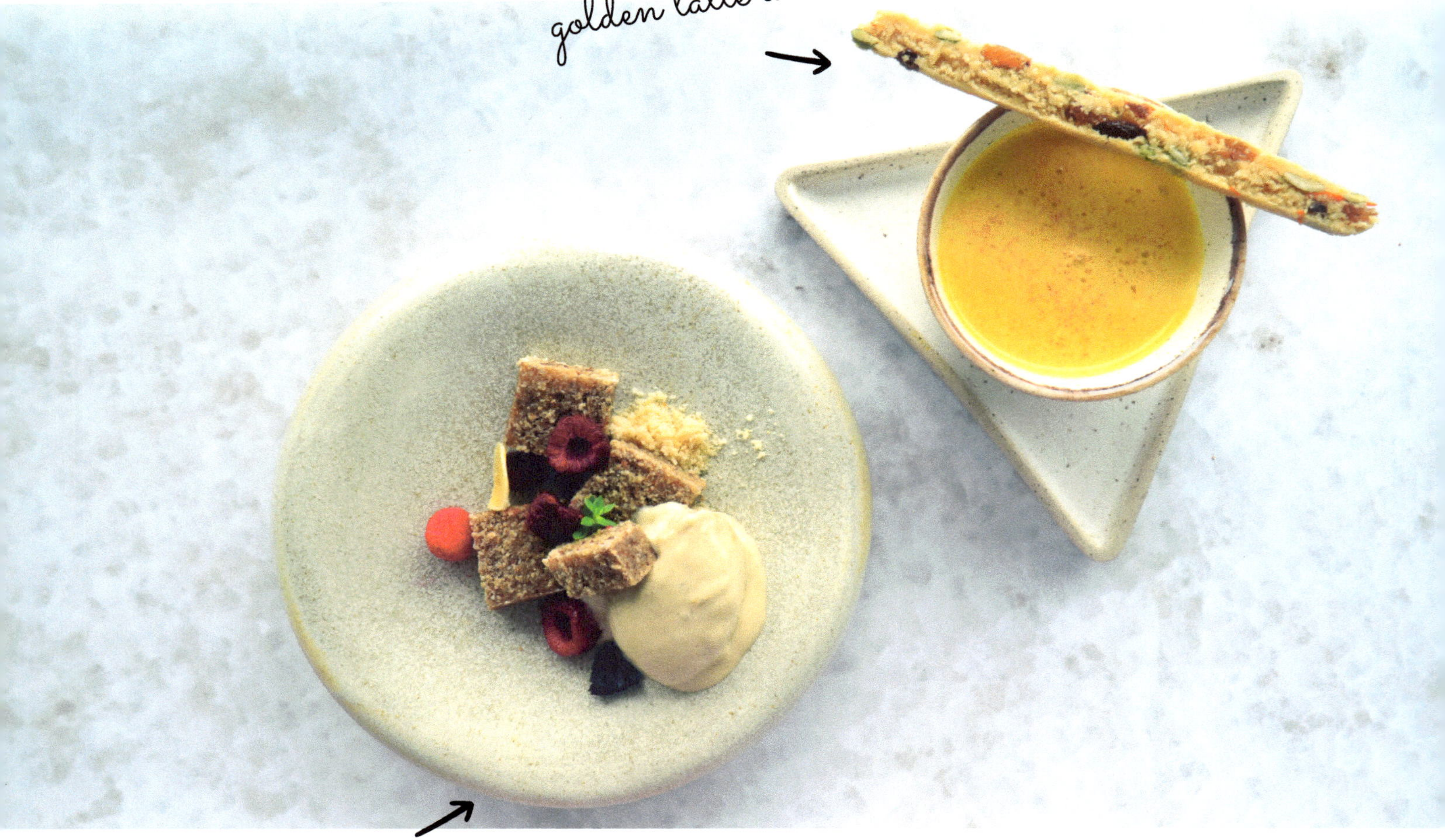

banana bread, icecream and berries

The State of Everything

INTRO

Best food is not only about the food you consume, also about the experience that you create. First, the components all play a roll in the overall dish and they are very important for the whole experience. Experimental flavors paired with crispy, jelly and creamy textures always make for a stellar experience. It is also very comprehensive, from the color of the plate you choose to its design, to the preparation stage, to its presentation, to the feelings you affect while preparing it. Details heighten our enjoyment of food and bring us into the present moment.

This book is pushing boundaries and reinventing raw vegan cuisine with the combination of raw cooking techniques. Besides dehydrated-raw and sous vide-raw, you will also find pure-raw recipes that do not require any special techniques to create the dishes.

Even if preparing raw dishes are super simple, knowing how to make a balanced and advanced one is not that straightforward. It takes an expert to arrange food in a way that makes the scents, aromas and flavors emerge. Combining the right ingredients and techniques is one of the most important things when it comes to having a fantastic eating experience and feeling good!

Food, in itself, doesn't always look as good as it could or should, it needs a little help from someone who truly loves it. When it's done right, plating creates its own kind of magic. In this book, you will learn how to make colors pop and how to make every ingredient look their best.
"Mad About Raw" inspires you to prepare raw foods in a contemporary, artistic manner utilizing the best ingredients!
Whether you are a restaurateur or an individual who wants to elevate raw eating experience and just get some inspiration, we strongly believe that the innovative ideas in this book will bring some magic to your life.

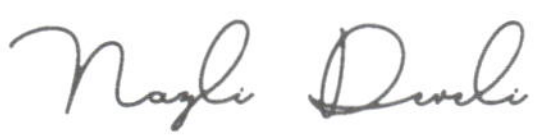

MAD ABOUT RAW

Food Designer, Chef & Author

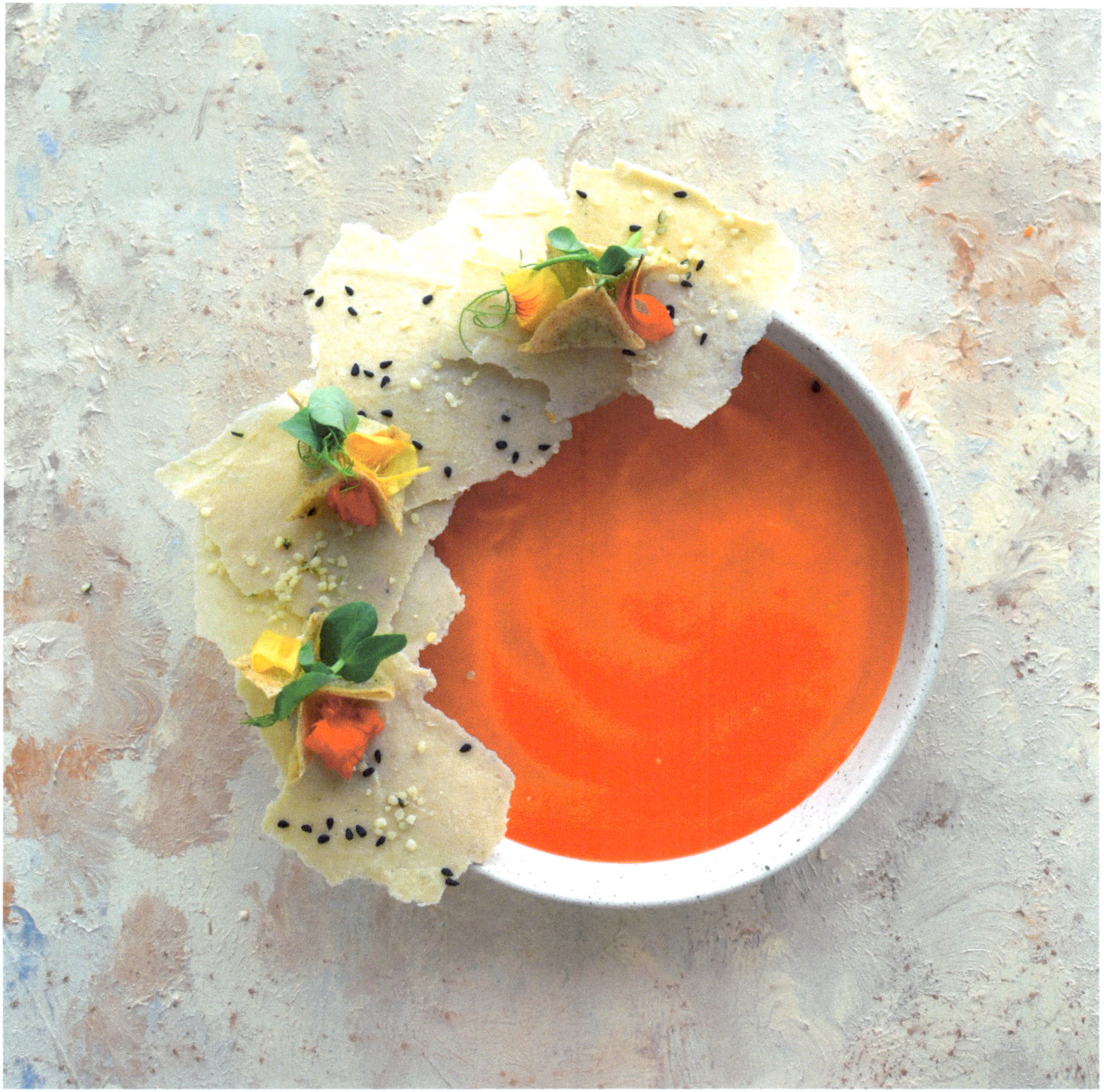

OVERVIEW TO RAW COOKING METHODS

Pure-Raw

Pure-Raw recipes usually don't use any special technique such as sous vide or dehydration to make them. They are easy to make recipes in minutes. Pure-raw recipes may require some easy techniques such as marination, fermentation, blending, sprouting, juicing and some equipments such as a spiralizer, mandolin slicer, food processor, blender.

Marination is the process of soaking foods in a seasoned, often acidic, liquid to add flavour to the dish. The basic ingredients of any marinade are salt , vinegar, herbs and oil.

Mandoline slicer is useful for getting perfectly even cuts, especially when you're trying to make them extra thin. It is part of every working chef's toolbox. Sure, a sharp knife will do the trick, but mandolines guarantee perfection and uniformity.

Spiralizers turn fresh veggies into faux-noodles. There are a few vegetables such as courgette, cucumber and root veggies that were born to be spiralized.

PS: Although fermenting is a big food trend these days, the author mostly avoids fermented foods. You'll find nothing but some gourmet touches with some fermented ingredients added in small amounts in this book.

Dehydrated-Raw

It means that the recipe is made in the food dehydrator - also known as raw food oven. A food is considered raw if it has never been heated over 40–46°C. It should also not be refined, pasteurized, treated with pesticides or otherwise processed in any way.

If you don't have a dehydrator, you can dehydrate in a convection oven too. But it will not be raw. Set the temperature about 50-60° C. For more air circulation you can keep oven door open (experiment with propping it open with a wood spoon). This is just an alternative suggestion but we cannot guarantee the same result. It is always best to make raw food recipes in the food dehydrator.
Recommended brand: Excalibur

Sous Vide-Raw

Sous Vide-Raw in this book means that the recipe is made with sous vide cooking technique. It's a method that involves vacuum-sealing food in a bag and cooking it in a water bath for several hours at a low temperature.

Raw food eaters can enjoy sous vide cooking, because the water can be heated to exactly 46° C. Food can easily be hot and raw at the same time, without being depleted of nutrients.

The key is to carefully monitor the heat to gently bring your food to the right temperature without overcooking it. Cooking in a bag locks in the food's natural juices, aroma and moisture, also reduces the effects of oxidation, so the color remains vibrant. This results in super-flavorful, ultra-tender and juicy. No matter what you cook, you'll love the flavor of a good sous vide.
Recommended brand: Tribest Sousvant + Stasher Premium Reusable Sous Vide Bags

If you don't have a sous vide machine, you can adjust the temperature of the water as needed. Here are the steps:

1. Fill a large, heavy-bottomed pot with as much water as you can without it overflowing when you add your food.
2. Bring the water to 46° C. You'll need to play with your heat settings to get it right. It takes a little trial and error to achieve a steady cooking temperature depending on your stove. We use Electrolux induction stove, when set it at 2, it allows to boil around 42° C.
3. Place your ingredients into reusable zip-close bags.
4. Make sure the ingredients are already cut into individual servings. Don't put too many pieces of food together into one bag. The ingredients need some room to move.
5. Place the bagged ingredients into the pot of heated water to cook.
6. Keep monitoring your temperature. As with heating the water, you want to keep it within 2° C of your ideal. Don't be afraid to remove it from the heat if it goes to high, but do keep an eye on it, and put it back on when it dips (not lower than 2° C below the ideal temperature). If it goes too high or too low for a bit, don't panic; just keep bringing it back to where you need it.

breakfast

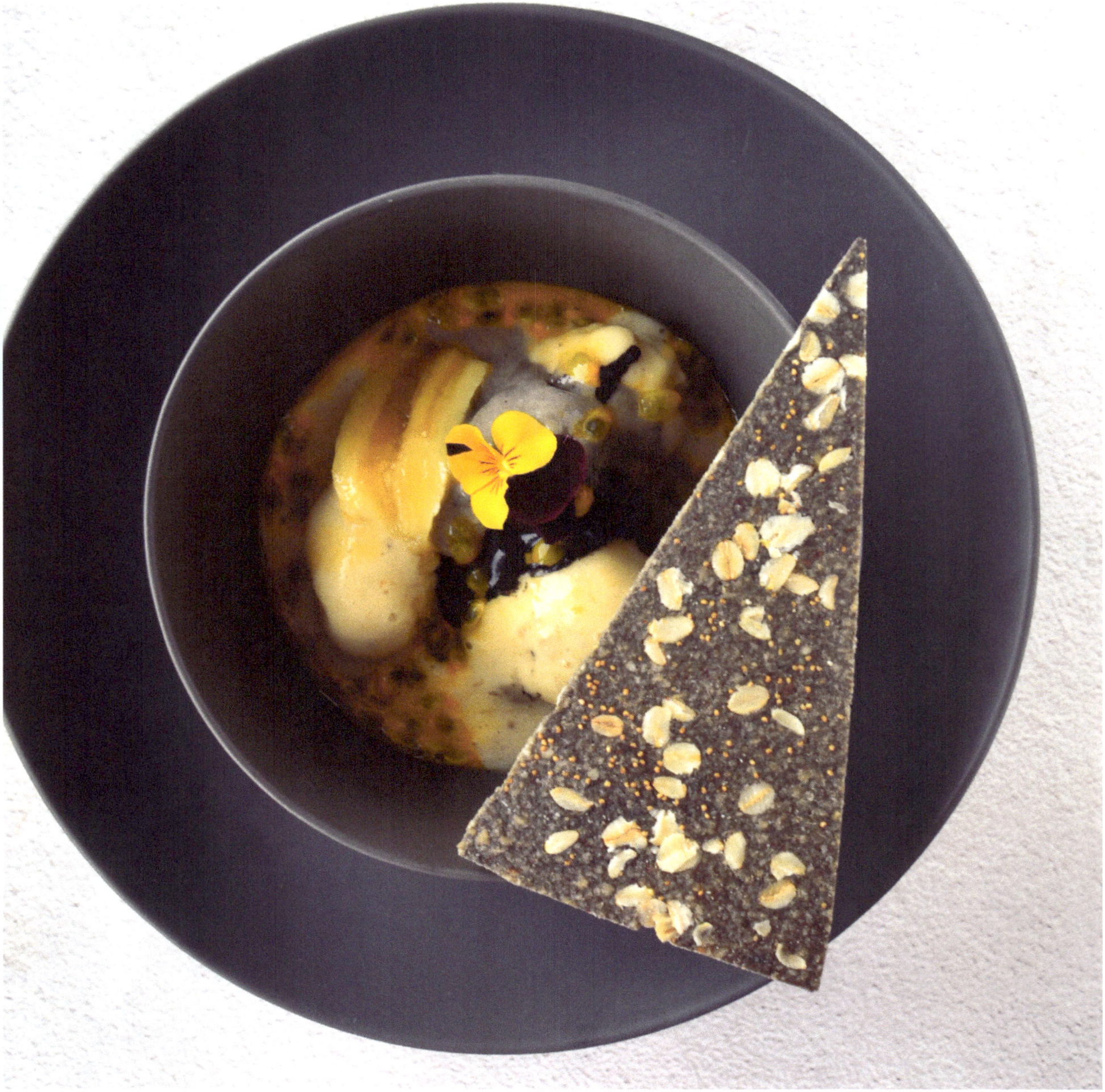

WANDERING STAR NICE CREAM

Category - Pure-Raw
Preperation - 10 minutes
Serves - 1-2 person

Equipment - Blender, Ice cream scooper
Personal note - Tropical feelings in winter

Nice cream ingredients

2 large semi-frozen banana
1 fresh banana
1 frozen peach
1 passion fruit
2 tbsp black tahini

Optional Add-On's

1 tsp maca powder
1 tbsp grated fresh ginger
1/4 tsp licorice salt (from Saltverk Iceland)

Instructions

1. To make nice cream, place the frozen bananas, peach and fresh bananas at room temperature into your blender. (If you will use optional add-on's, add all of them at this stage.) Blend on batter mode if you are using Blendtec until smooth and thick but not too liquid. Avoid blending too much.
2. Once done, using an icecream scooper, scoop 2 balls from the mixture, place into your bowl.
3. Then add 1 tbsp black tahini into your blender, blend until you get gray color.
4. Using the ice cream scooper, transfer a ball to your bowl.
5. Drizzle 1 tbsp tahini over the nice cream.
6. Add 1/2 passion fruit and a piece of thinly sliced banana.
7. Serve with oatmeal thins if desired. These thins also can be eaten as they are. See the oatmeal thins recipe on the next page.

OATMEAL THINS

Category - Dehydrated-Raw
Dehydration time - 6 hours
Makes - 30x30 cm dehydrator tray

Equipment - Food processor, dehydrator and spatula
Personal note - A satisfying raw food experience in winter days

Oat thin ingredients

240 g gluten free sprouted rolled oats
75 g dried raisins
80 g almond flour
3 tbsp coconut oil
3 tbsp black tahini
3 tbsp maple syrup or coconut nectar
2 tbsp psyllium husk powder
50 ml water
A pinch salt
Yellow poppy seeds to sprinkle
1 tsp activated charcoal (optional to get light black color)

Instructions

1. Soak the sprouted rolled oats and dried raisins in warm water for 5 minutes then strain and drain, transfer to your food processor.
2. Add the almond flour, psyllium husk powder, water, salt, maple, charcoal, black tahini and coconut oil. Blend well until you get a dough texture.
3. Spread mixture on a parchment paper. Put another parchment paper on the top. Using a rolling pin, gently roll the dough out, flatten out as much as possible. Once done, remove the parchment paper. Sprinkle some yellow poppy seeds and rolled oats on top.
4. Bake at 42° C in the dehydrator for 6 hours then flip up and continue baking for 2-3 hours or until get desired crispy texture.
5. Once baked, transfer it to your cutting board. Using a sharp chef knife, cut the thins into triangle or desired shape. Serve with your nice cream or enjoy as it is.

GINGERBREAD SMOOTHIE

Category - Pure-Raw
Preperation - 6 minutes
Serves - 2 person

Equipment - Blender, tea strainer
Personal note - Very festive!

Ingredients
3 large semi-frozen banana
100 ml coconut milk
1 small semi-frozen red apple
1/2 tsp gingerbread spice
1 tsp vanilla bean powder
2 tbsp almond butter
Cinnamon powder to dust

Instructions
1. Combine all ingredients in a high-power blender, blend until smooth.
2. Transfer mixture into your bowl.
3. You'll want to sift the cinnamon powder for a nice even layer without clumps, but if you don't have a dedicated flour or sugar sifter, use a tea strainer to get the same effect.
4. Serve with gingerbread men cookies if desired. See the gingerbread men cookie recipe on the next page.

Notes: You can substitute bananas with cauliflower, mango, pineapple or young coconut meat. But for the best tasting smoothie, recommended to use the ripe bananas.

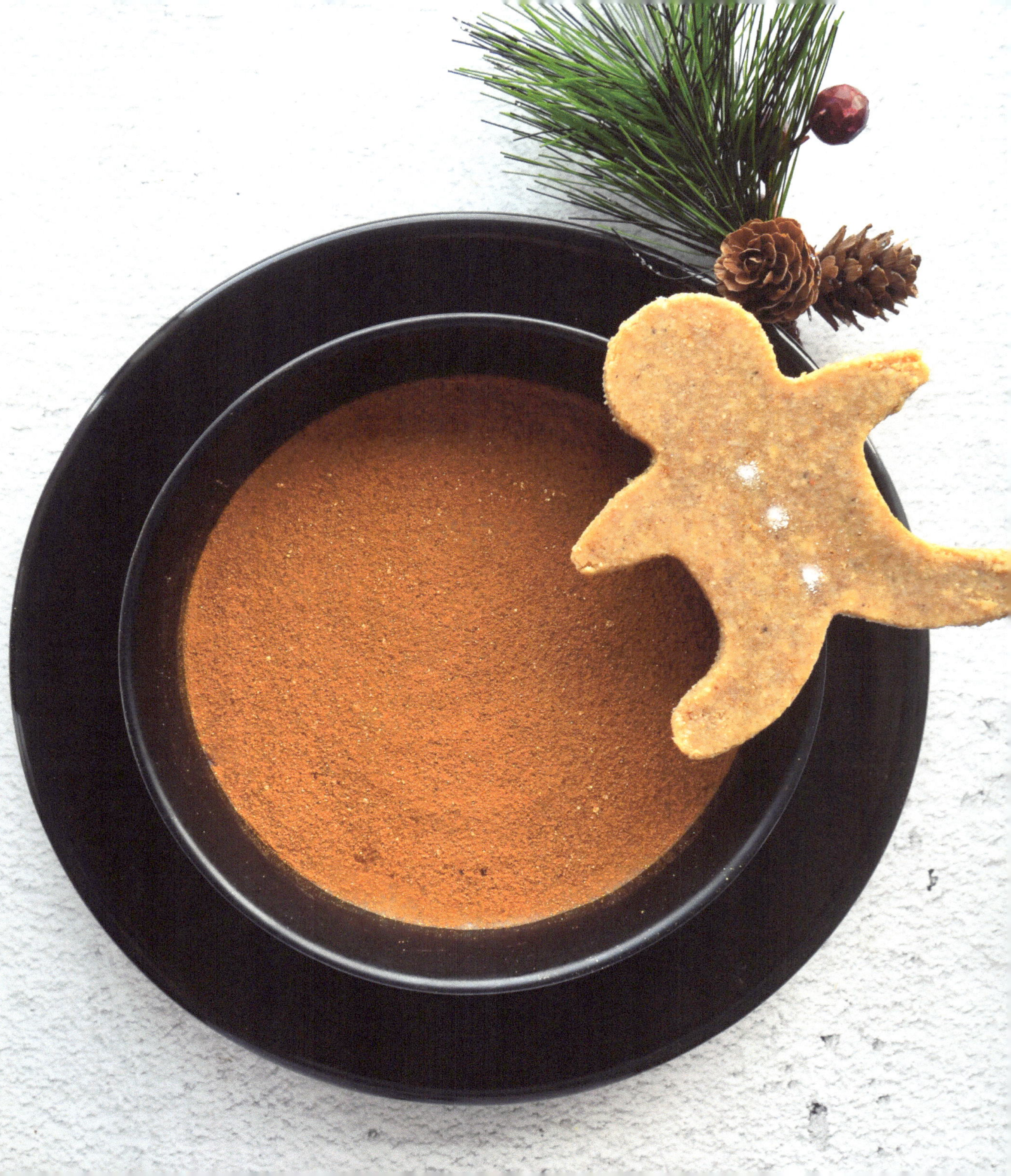

GINGERBREAD MEN COOKIES

Category - Dehydrated-Raw
Dehydration - Approx. 10 hours
Makes - 7-8 cookies

Equipment - Food processor, dehydrator, gingermen cookie cutter

Ingredients

1 + 1/2 cup almond flour
1/2 cup coconut flour
2 tbsp psyllium husk powder
6 tbsp coconut milk
4 tbsp coconut sugar powdered
2 tbsp maple syrup
1 tbsp coconut oil
1/2 tsp ginger powder
1/2 tsp cinnamon powder
1/8 tsp clove powder
1/8 tsp nutmeg powder
1/4 tsp pink himalayan salt

Instructions

1. Place dry ingredients; almond flour, coconut flour, psyllium powder, coconut sugar (grind in the coffee grinder first), ginger, cinnamon, clove, nutmeg and salt to your food processor. Blend until well combined.
2. Then add the maple syrup, melted coconut oil and coconut milk and thoroughly incorporate.
3. Ball up the dough with your hands and place on a non-stick dehydrator sheet. Take another non-stick sheet and place on the dough. Flatten the cookie dough by pressing down firmly, by using a rolling pin roll over between the dehydrator sheets until about 3-6mm thick. Remove the sheet from the top.
4. Using a gingerbread cookie cutter, shape your dough. Remove the edges of the dough. Repeat the process for the rest of the dough.
5. Dehydrate for 3 hours at 46° C, then flip the cookie sheet over another tray, remove the non-stick sheet.
6. Allow to dehydrate them at 38° C until crispy. It usually takes between 8-10 hours.
7. Serve with your gingerbread nice cream or eat as it is.

CHOCOLATE CEREAL

Category - Dehydrated-Raw
Dehydration time - 8 hrs
Sprouting time - 36-48 hrs
Serves - 4-6 person

Equipment - Food processor, dehydrator
Storage - In the airtight container up to 2-3 weeks

Ingredients

2 cups sprouted buckwheat soaked
100 g maple syrup
2 tbsp raw cacao powder
1/2 tsp maca powder
A pinch of salt

Add-on's:

1 + 1/2 cup plant milk
1/2 cup sliced bananas
2 tbsp forest berries

Instructions

1. Soak raw buckwheat groats in the water for 30-40 minutes, rinse a few times and let it sit in an open top jar, laying the jar on its side (or put a strainer to hold it under turn bottom upside, to contact with more air-buckwheat particules) rinse everyday and let it sit, you have sprouts in about 36-48 hours. Once sprouted, transfer them to your food processor.
2. Add the maple syrup, raw cacao powder, maca powder and salt.
3. Process until combined but not completely pureed.
4. Divide mixture between silicon lined dehydrator trays and spread to about 3mm thickness.
5. Dehydrate at 46° C for 6-7 hours or until completely dried.
6. You may need to flip it and continue to dehydrate additional 1-2 hours until completely crispy.
7. Once done, break into pieces. They are ready to eat!
8. Serve with bananas, fresh forest fruits and nut milk if desired.

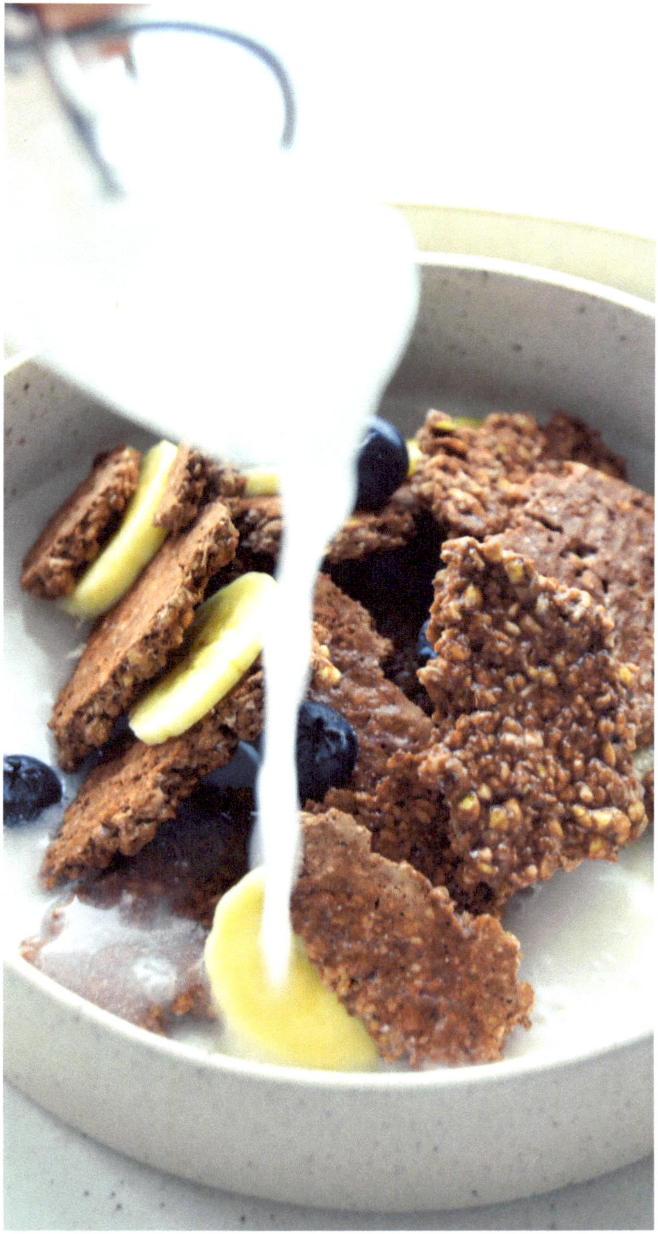

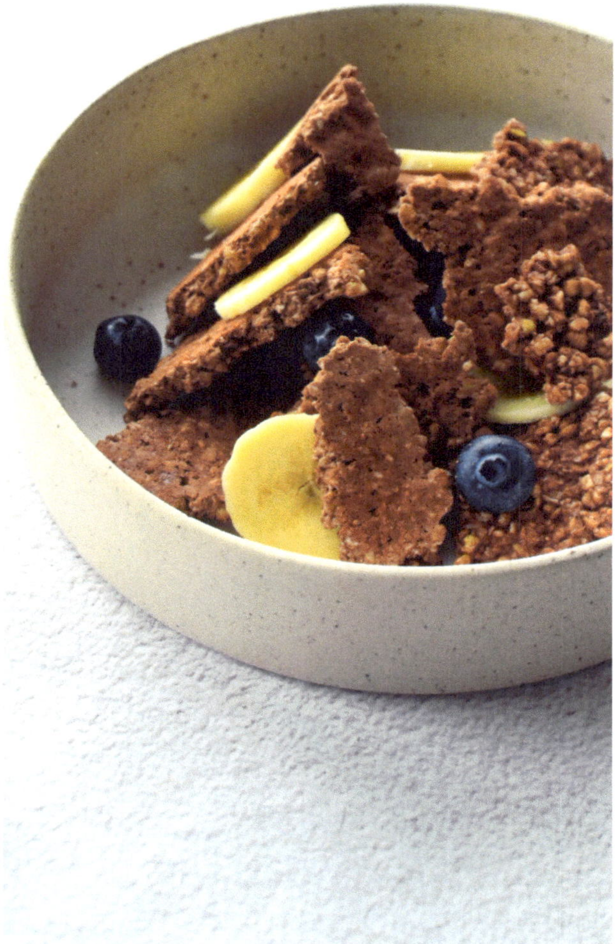

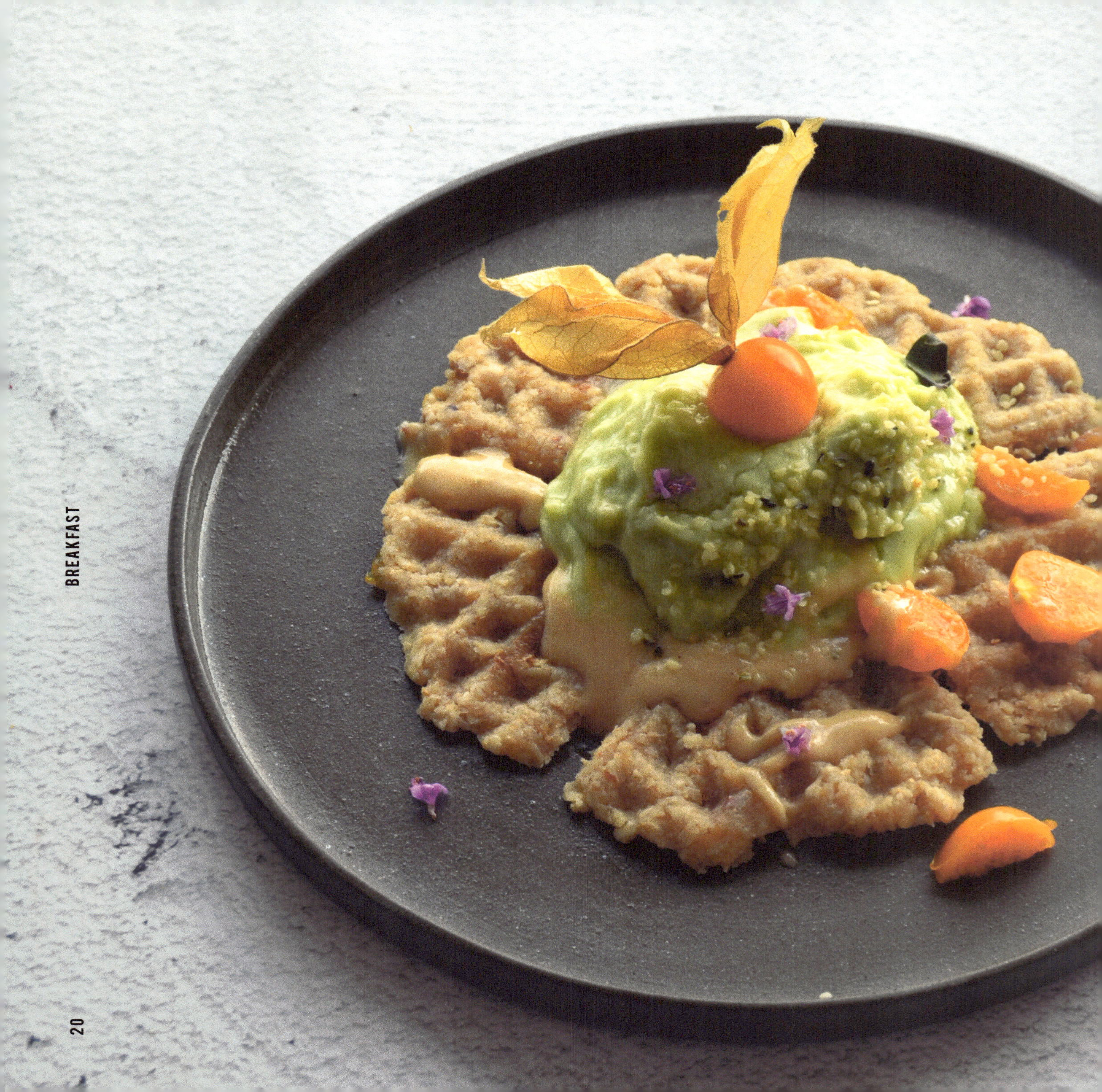

OAT WAFFLES

Category - Dehydrated-Raw
Dehydration time - 8 hours
Quantity - 4 whole waffles

Storage- In the fridge, up to 7 days
Equipments - Food processor, dehydrator, waffle shape mould or waffle maker to shape it.

Ingredients

240 g gluten-free sprouted oatmeal
75 g dried raisins
80 g almond flour
3 tbsp coconut oil
3 tbsp maple or coconut nectar syrup
2 tbsp psyllium husk powder
150 ml water
1/4 tsp licorice salt (from Saltverk Iceland)

Instructions

1. Soak the rolled sprouted oats and dried raisins in warm water for 5 minutes then strain, drain and transfer to your food processor.
2. Add the almond flour, psyllium husk powder, water, salt, maple and coconut oil. Blend well until you get a dough texture.
3. Spread mixture on a parchment paper or non stick silicon dehydrator sheets. Place another parchment paper on it, using a rolling pin gently roll the dough out, flatten out as much as possible.
4. Then transfer it to a waffle mould or alternatively you can use waffle maker with lined cling film (Do not turn on waffle maker, we wil use it for waffle-shaping only). Press for 10-15 seconds to shape. Then remove from the waffle machine.
5. Trim off the edges so it looks nicer.
6. Carefully open waffle maker and remove each waffle and place onto dehydrator mesh tray.
7. Bake at 42° C for 5-6 hours then flip up and continue baking for 2-3 hours or until get desired chewy texture. Serve with nut butters, avocado ice cream, your favorite fruits or whatever you like!

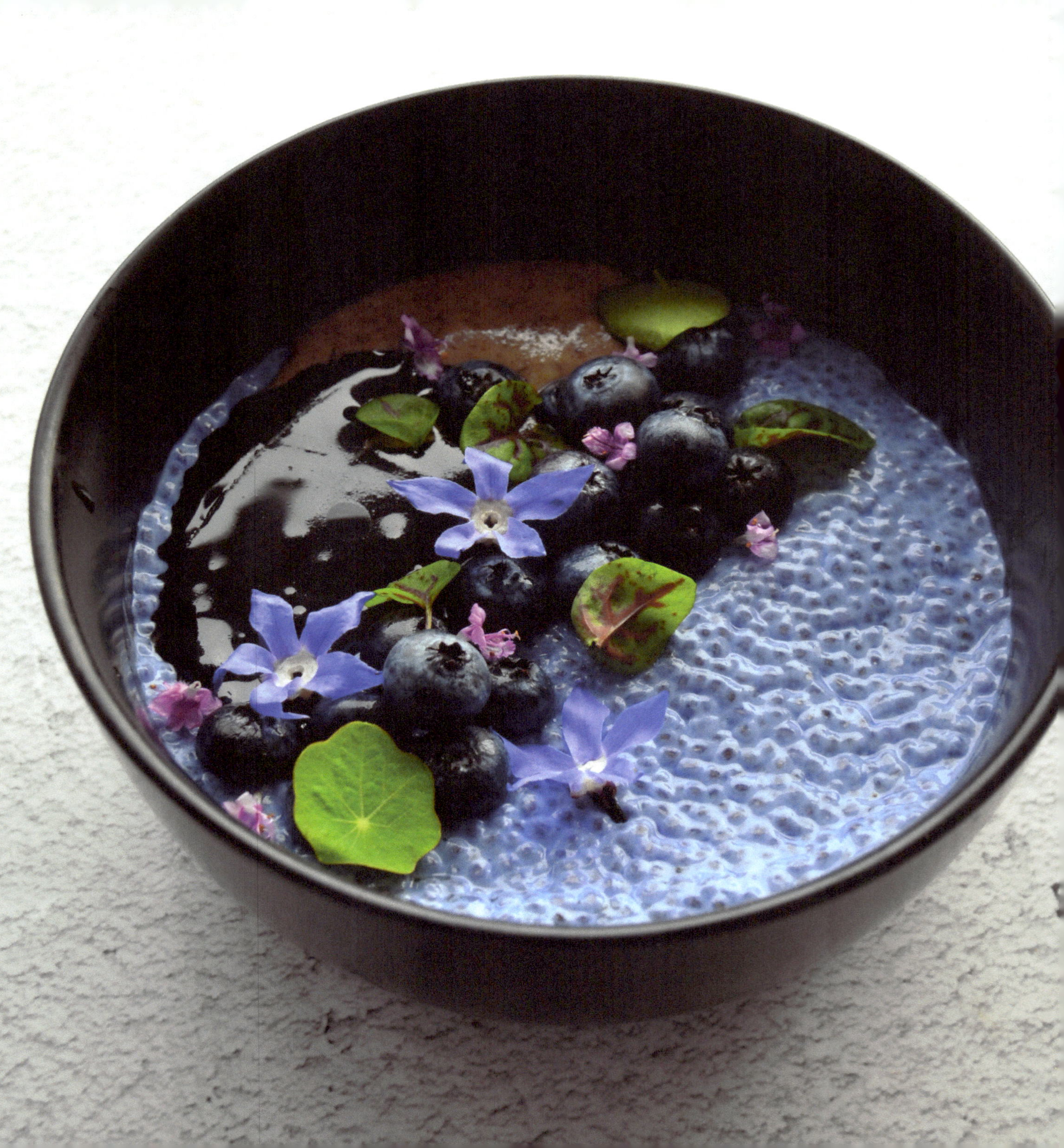

SKY CHIA PUDDING

Category - Pure-Raw
Preperation - 5 min + 30 min setting
Quantity - 2 person

Equipment - A mason jar
Storage: up to 3 days in an airtight container in the refrigerator.
Personal note - Omega-3 source

Ingredients
3 tbsp chia seeds
2 tbsp butterfly pea flower powder
300 ml coconut milk
2 tbsp almond butter
1 tbsp black tahini (optional)
1 tbsp maple syrup

to decorate:
nasturtium leaves
vene cress
borage
purple basil flower
blueberries

Instructions
1. Place the chia seeds, maple syrup, butterfly pea flower powder in a jar. Add the coconut milk. Close the lid of the jar. Shake well until butterfly pea flower powder dissolves completely.
2. Once the chia pudding mixture is well combined, let it sit for 5 minutes, give it another shake to break up any clumps of chia seeds, cover and put the mixture in the fridge to set for 1-2 hours or overnight. The chia pudding should be nice and thick, not liquidy. If it's not thick enough, just add more chia seeds (about 1 tbsp), stir and refrigerate for another 30 minutes or so.
3. Open the lid of your jar, place chia pudding in a bowl, add some almond butter and black tahini on top.
4. Serve with fresh blueberries and decorate with borage, nasturtium leaves , vene cress and borage if desired.

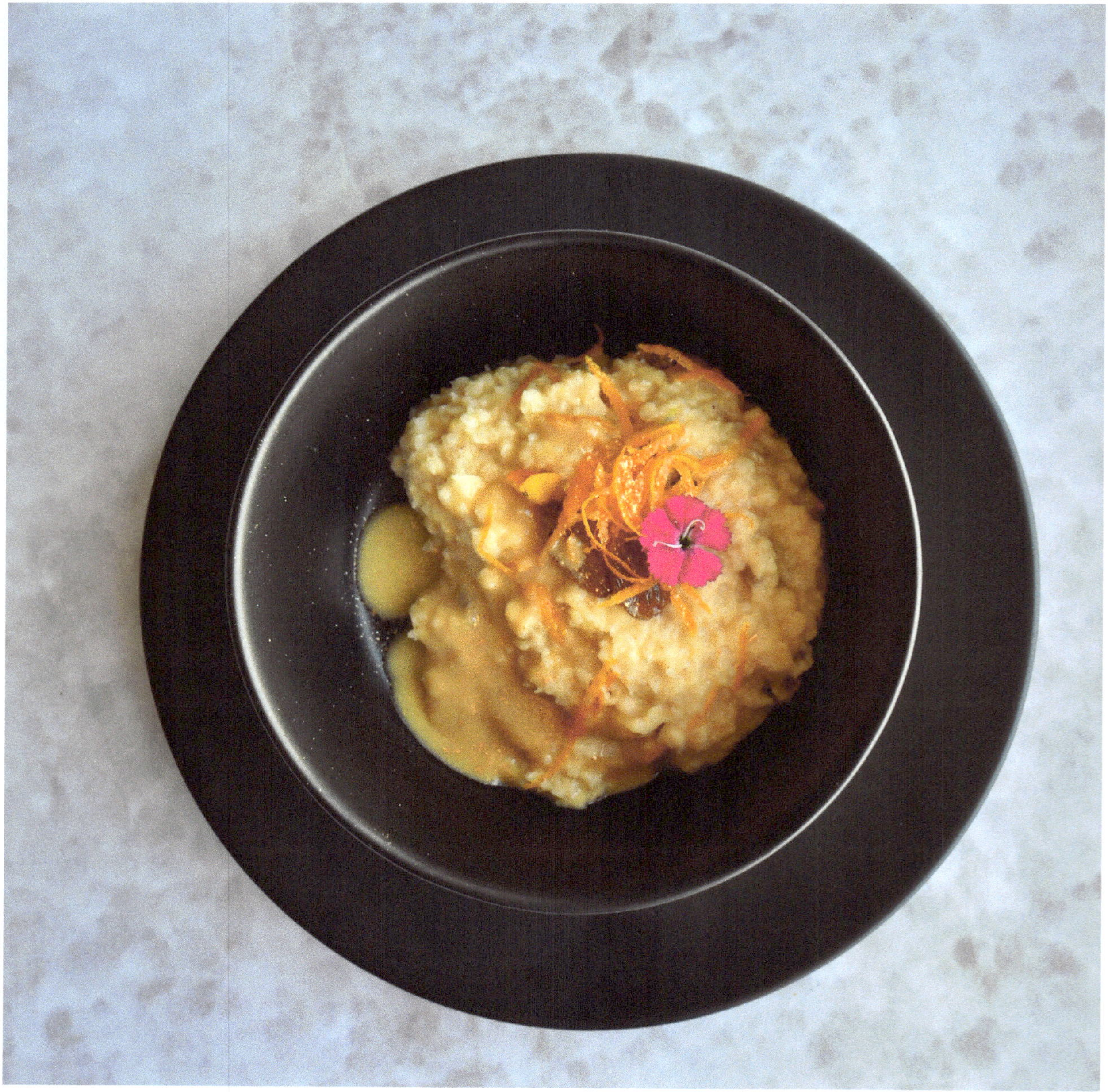

KOHLRABI PORRIDGE

Category - Pure-Raw
Preperation - 15 minutes
Quantity - 2 person

Equipment - High speed blender
Personal note - An exciting new experience!

Ingredients
130 g kohlrabi
50 g almond butter
60 ml fresh orange juice
1 tbsp maple syrup
1/8 tsp cardamom
1 tsp cinnamon
1/4 tsp vanilla powder
1/4 tsp freshly grated ginger
A pinch of salt

Instructions
1. Peel the kohlrabi and cut it into chunks around 1" wide.
2. Blend the kohlrabi pieces in a food processor until they break down to look rice-like. Squeeze out the excess water.
3. Pour almond butter over the riced kohlrabi. Using a spoon, mix well.
4. Blend up the orange juice, maple, cinnamon, cardamom, vanilla, ginger and a pinch of salt in the blender until smooth. Pour over the riced kohlrabi. Combine well.
5. Transfer mixture in a large bowl.
6. Finely peel the orange, put orange zest on your bowl, along with the raisins. Dust some cinnamon powder if desired. Enjoy.

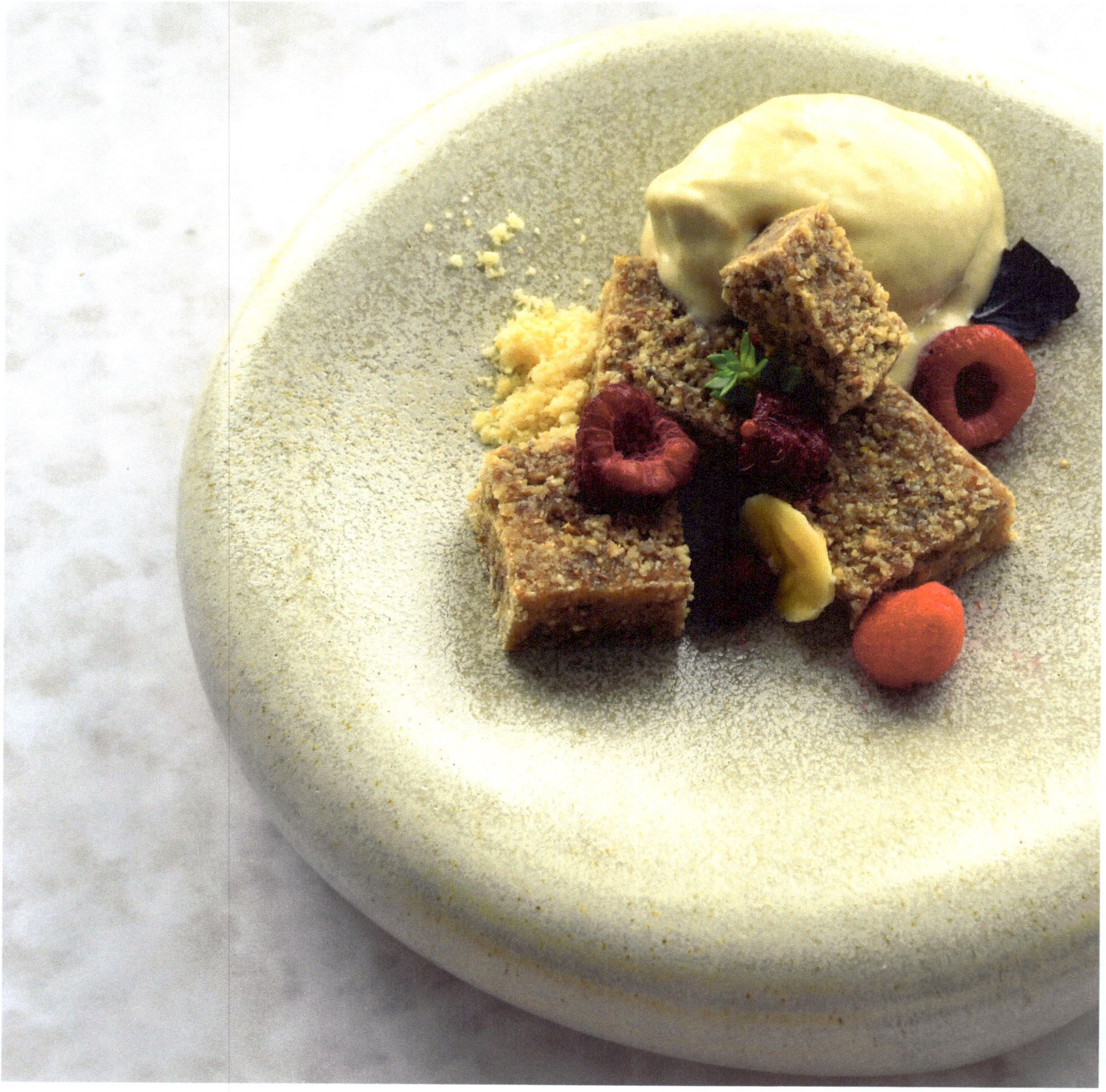

BANANA BREAD WITH TAHINI ICE CREAM

Category - Dehydrated-Raw
Preperation - 20 min + 4 hrs dehydration
Quantity - 4-6 person

Equipment - Coffee grinder, dehydrator, 20x8 cm loaf tin, mixing bowl
Personal note - balances you on so many levels!

Banana Bread Ingredients

2.5 cups rolled oats
1 cup almond flour
1/2 cup flaxseed
1 tbsp chia seeds
3 large bananas
1/2 cup maple syrup
1 tsp vanilla extract
1/4 cup almond milk
1/2 tsp salt

Instructions

1. Process the oats, almond flour, and flax seed into flour either together or separately, depending on the equipment. Coffee grinder works best.
2. Add all of the ingredients to a mixing bowl, mash the bananas, and lightly fold everything together.
3. Form a loaf in the loaf tin and place it on the dehydrator tray with the tin.
4. Dehydrate at 46° C for 1-2 hours until crust forms on the outside. Once the bread is firm enough, remove from the tin, slice it. Place the slices on the silicon sheets.
5. Dehydrate slices at 42° C for another 3-4 hours or until completely dried.

Serve immediately or keep in the refrigerator. Just heat in the dehydrator before eating.
Check the next page to see the other components of this dish.

banana bread continued

TAHINI ICE CREAM

Category - Pure-Raw
Time: 7-8 minutes
Makes - 1 cup

Equipment - High speed blender, ice cream scoop
Personal note - Verstaile!

Ingredients

3 large frozen bananas
3 tbsp unroasted tahini
1/2 tbsp psyllium husk powder
A pinch of licorice salt

Instructions

1. Place all the ingredients to your blender.
2. Blend until smooth but thick nice cream mixture.

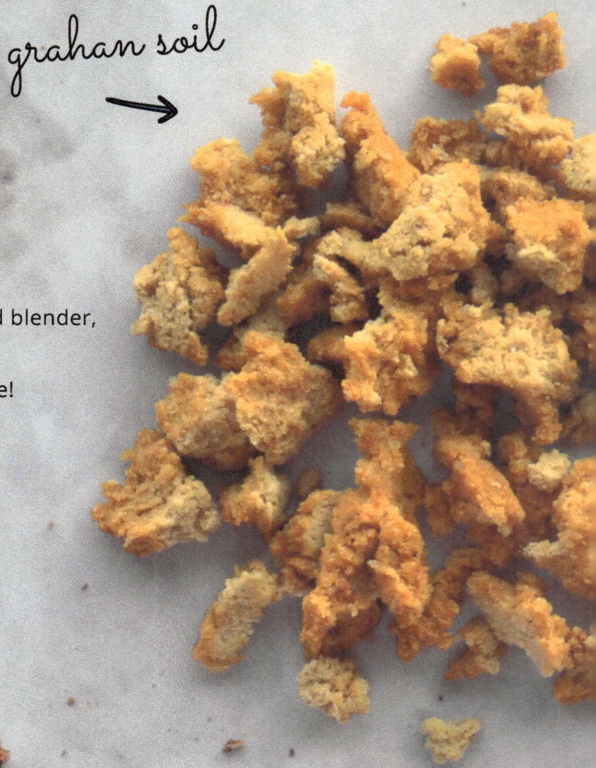

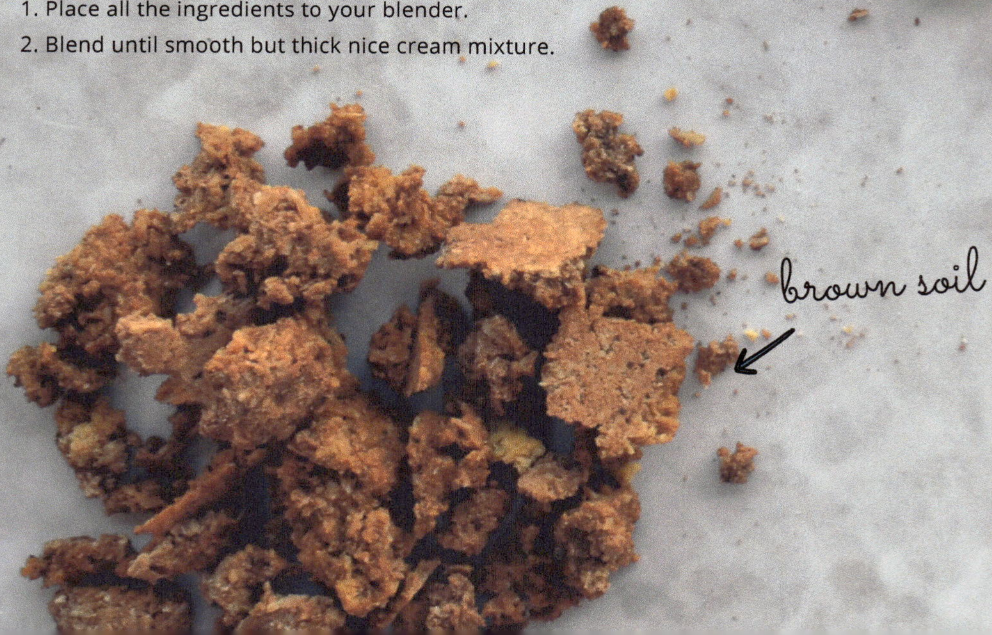

banana bread continued

ALMOND SOIL TYPES

Category - Dehydrated-Raw
Dehydration time: 8 hrs
Makes - 1 cup

Equipment - food processor, dehydrator
Personal note - Verstaile!

Ingredients

120 g almond milk pulp wet
50 g desiccated coconut
50 g coconut sugar for the graham soil (use agave for white soil, use raw cacao or carob for brown soil)
1/2 tsp pink himalayan salt

Instructions

Mix all the ingredients together. Place the mixture onto a dehydrator sheet, allowing some of the mixture to form large clumps. You want to combine this variety of textures in your dish. Dehydrate at 42° C overnight or 6-8 hours, until completely dried and crispy enough.

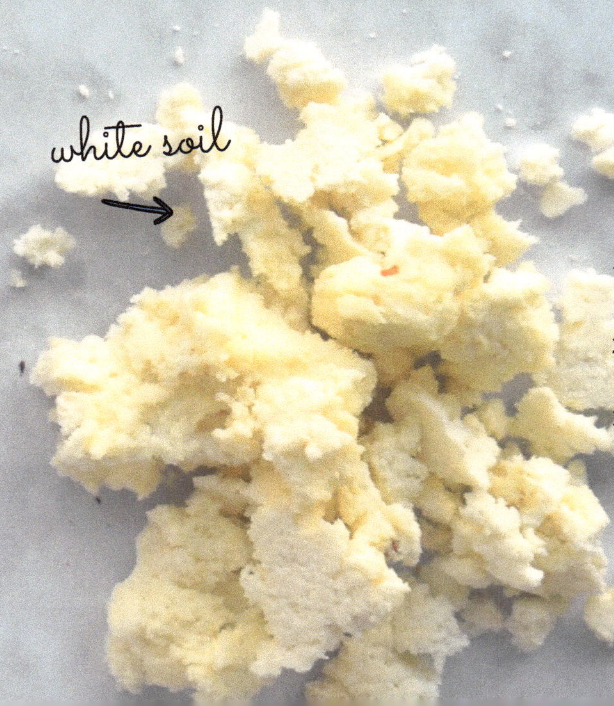

Decoration

Raspberries, sliced bananas, fresh basil

Assembly

1. Cut your banana bread in small squares. Place into the plate.
2. Add 1 tbsp almond soil. If you want fine soil, blend the soil in the food processor before using.
3. Using an ice cream scoop, scoop a ball from the tahini icre cream. Place on the banana bread.
4. Add fresh raspberries and sliced bananas.
5. Garnish with fresh basil. Enjoy!

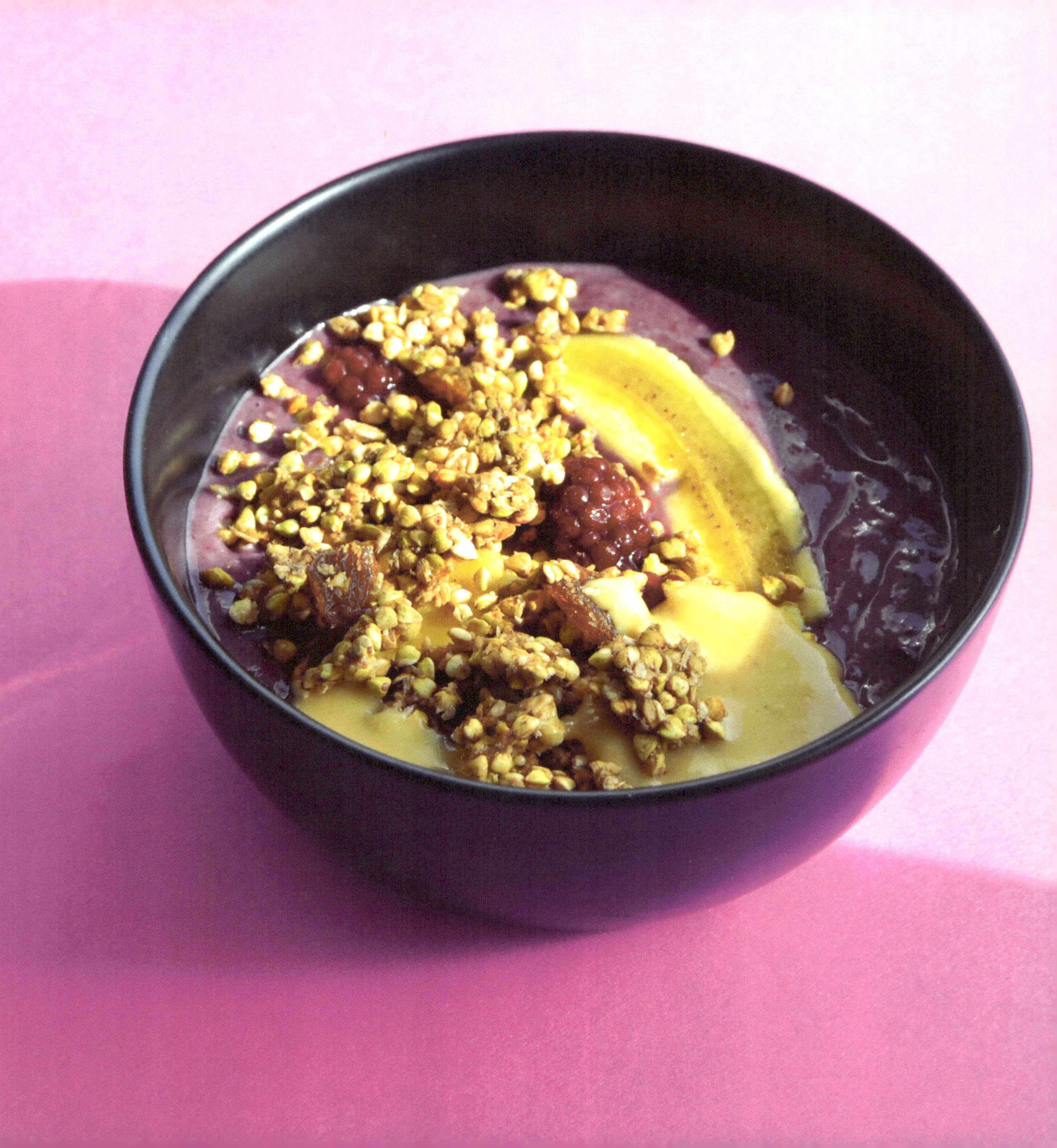

GINGERBREAD BUCKWHEAT RAWNOLA

Category - Dehydrated- Raw
Preperation - 20 mins + 5 hrs dehydration
Quantity - 2-4 person

Equipment - Food processor, dehydrator
Note- Oil-free, sugar-free

Rawnola ingredients

2 cups raw buckwheat groats
2 large mashed ripe bananas
1 tsp cinnamon
1/4 tsp cardamom
1/4 tsp ground ginger
1/2 cup dried raisins soaked
1 tsp licorice salt

Blackberry smoothie bowl

4 frozen bananas
1 cup frozen blackberries
1/2 tsp spirulina
1/2 tsp baobab powder
1 tbsp almond butter
Fresh sliced banana and blackberries

Instructions

1. Place buckwheat groats in a bowl, cover with water. Let it soak for 2 hours. Then wash, rinse and strain the excess water.
2. Add the mashed bananas (alternatively you can use fresh red apple puree), cinnamon, cardamom, ginger, soaked and strained raisins and licorice salt. Use your hands or a spatula to toss all the ingredients until all is coated. (This is oil and sugar free granola, you can also add 1 tbsp coconut oil + 2 tbsp coconut sugar if you prefer.)
3. Line a dehydrator tray with a non stick sheet and scatter the contents onto the sheet like you would granola. We want to encourage clusters to form, so don't separate the mixture too much. Allow small clumps to form. Dehydrate at 42° C for 4-5 hours then flip onto mesh and dry a further 5 hours or until crisp.
You can store in an air-tight jar in the room temperature for up to 4 weeks.
4. Place all the blackberry smoothie ingredients except fresh fruits and almond butter into your blender. Blend until well combined. Pour in a bowl. Add the sliced banana, blackberries and almond butter. Serve with the rawnola.

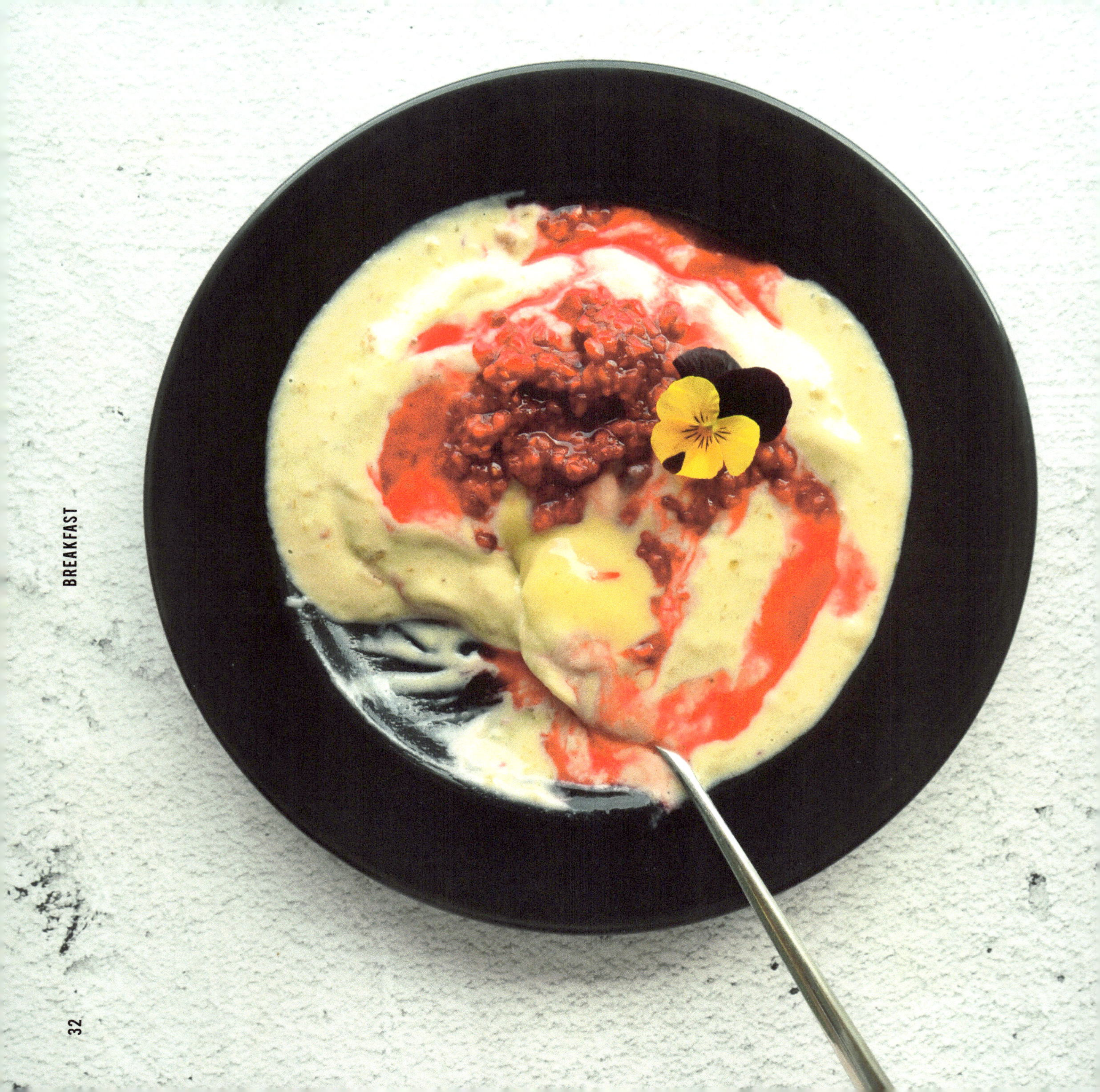

BANANA PEANUT SOFTSERVE

Category - Pure-Raw
Preperation - 6 minutes
Quantity - 2 person

Equipment - High speed blender
Personal note - Guilt-free pleasure!

Ingredients
3 large semi-frozen banana
2 tbsp peanut butter
1/4 tsp pink himalayan salt
Pansies to decorate

Raspberry coulis:
1/2 cup frozen raspberries
1 tbsp orange or lemon juice
1 tbsp maple syrup
1/4 tsp vanilla bean powder

Instructions
1. Combine the coulis ingredients in the Blendtec twister jar until the raspberries have broken down. If you want it to have a pourable consistency, blend a little longer.
2. Then using a strainer, strain the mixture. Remove the pulp. You can also use it without straining. This is how we love.
3. Place all the smoothie ingredients bananas, peanut butter and salt into your blender. Blend until smooth. Then transfer in a bowl.
4. Pour your coulis over the smoothie. Add additional peanut butter if desired. Decorate with yellow-brown pansies. Serve immediately!

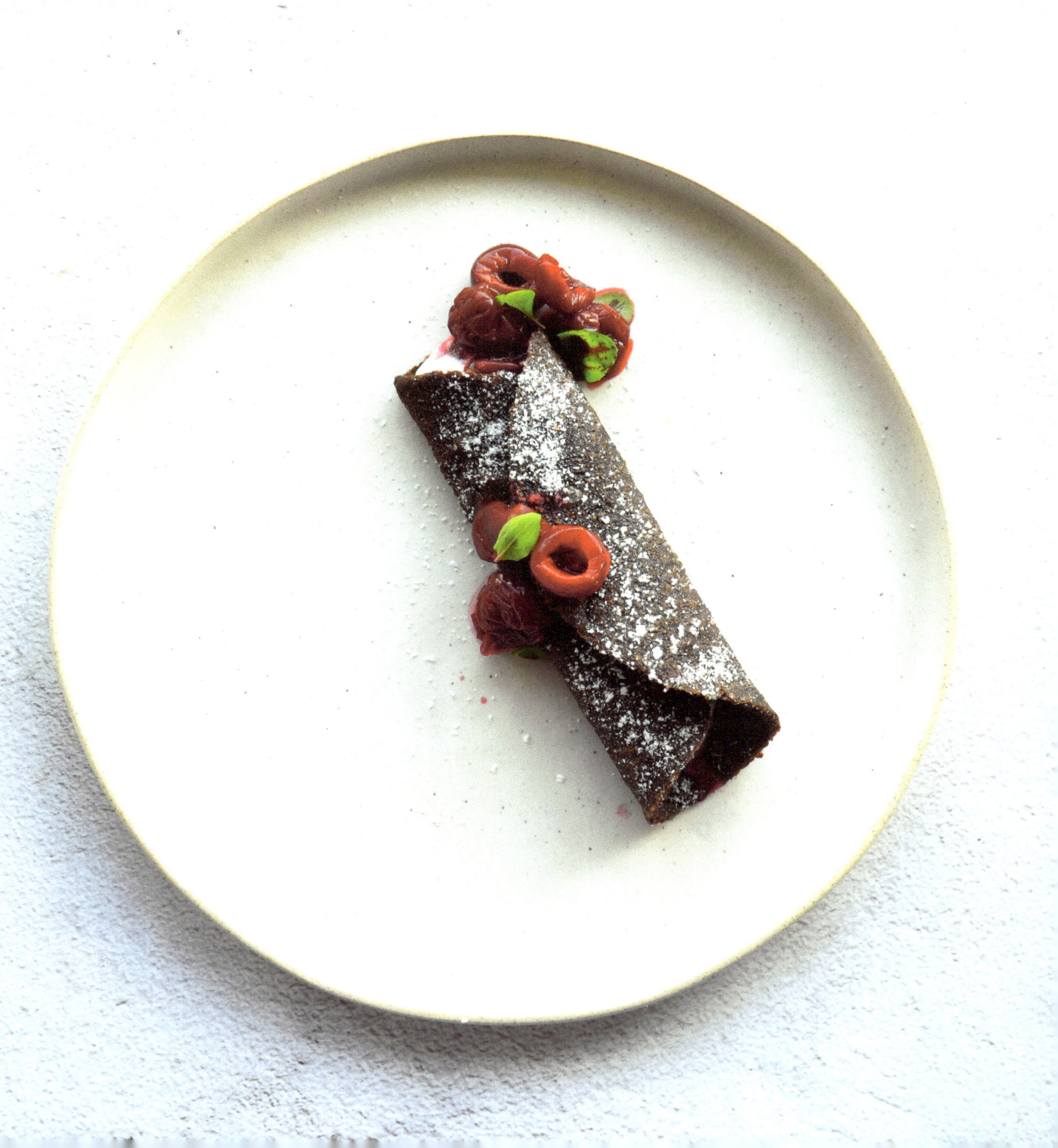

CHOCOLATE CRÊPES

Category - Dehydrated-Raw
Preperation - 4 hours
Quantity - 2 person

Equipment - Blender, dehydrator, spatula
Storage- Up to 5 days in an airtight contai-ner in the refrigerator.

Ingredients

60 g flaxseeds
2 tbsp chia seeds
250 g bananas
1 tbsp coconut sugar
1 tbsp raw cacao powder
1/2 tsp vanilla powder
1/4 tsp cinnamon powder
A pinch of salt

Instructions

1. Using a coffee grinder, grind chia , coconut sugar and flax seeds separately.
2. Place the bananas into your food processor. Blend until very smooth.
3. Then add the powdered coconut sugar, ground chia and flax meal. Blend again until smooth. The consistency should be that of pancake mixture.
4. Add the raw cacao powder, vanilla, cinnamon and a pinch of salt. Combine together.
5. Spread mixture onto the dehydrator sheets lined parchment paper. Bake at 42° C for 4 hrs.
6. Be careful and do not to over-dry the wraps. If the crêpes become too dry and start cracking around the edges, you can remedy the situation by dabbing a bit of water on the distressed areas, or trim off the edges when you cut the wraps up.

CRÊPE FILLING CREAM

Category - Pure-Raw
Time: 7-8 min prep + 4 hrs soaking
Makes - 1 cup

Equipment - High speed blender
Personal note - Verstaile!

Ingredients

1 cup macadamia
1/4 cup coconut milk
1 tsp vanilla extract or
1 vanilla bean powder
1 tbsp maple syrup
2 tbsp lemon juice
4-5 tbsp water

Instructions

1. In a blender add the soaked and strained macadamias (alternatively use cashews, almonds or young coconut meat), coconut milk, vanilla extract, maple (alternatively coconut nectar syrup), lemon juice (alternatively apple cider vinegar), and pinch salt.

2. Blend or pulse to combine. Then, slowly pour in a few tablespoons water until the mixture blends into a smooth, creamy and fluffy cream.

Other components

1/2 cup fresh or defrosted cherries

Erythritol or coconut flour for a snowy look

Assembly

1. Wash and dry your fruits.
2. Lay the crêpes on a work surface. Place macadamia cream in the centre of the wrap. Spread the mixture through the middle of the wrap so that almost reaches the edges.
2. Add the sliced fruits on to the macadamia cream, spread well.
3. Roll the crêpes tightly. Dust some erythritol over the plate to give a snowy look. Alternatively you can dust coconut flour. Enjoy!

Notes:

Storage: Crêpes can be made 1-2 days ahead. Cover and keep in fridge. When ready to eat, cover in foil and place in the dehydrator at 42° C for 45-50 minutes or until warm. Macadamia Cream can also be made ahead. It will keep in fridge for up to 3 days. It can also be frozen and defrosted. Allow 45 minutes to defrost.

Tips: Do not dehydrate crêpes overnight. The dehydrating time matters every bit as much as the recipe itself; if you over-dehydrate your crêpes, you'll end up either with brittle cracker. You have to check in on the crêpes during the dehydration process, test the texture, and make sure you're not letting things get too dry. They should be pliable, yet sturdy.

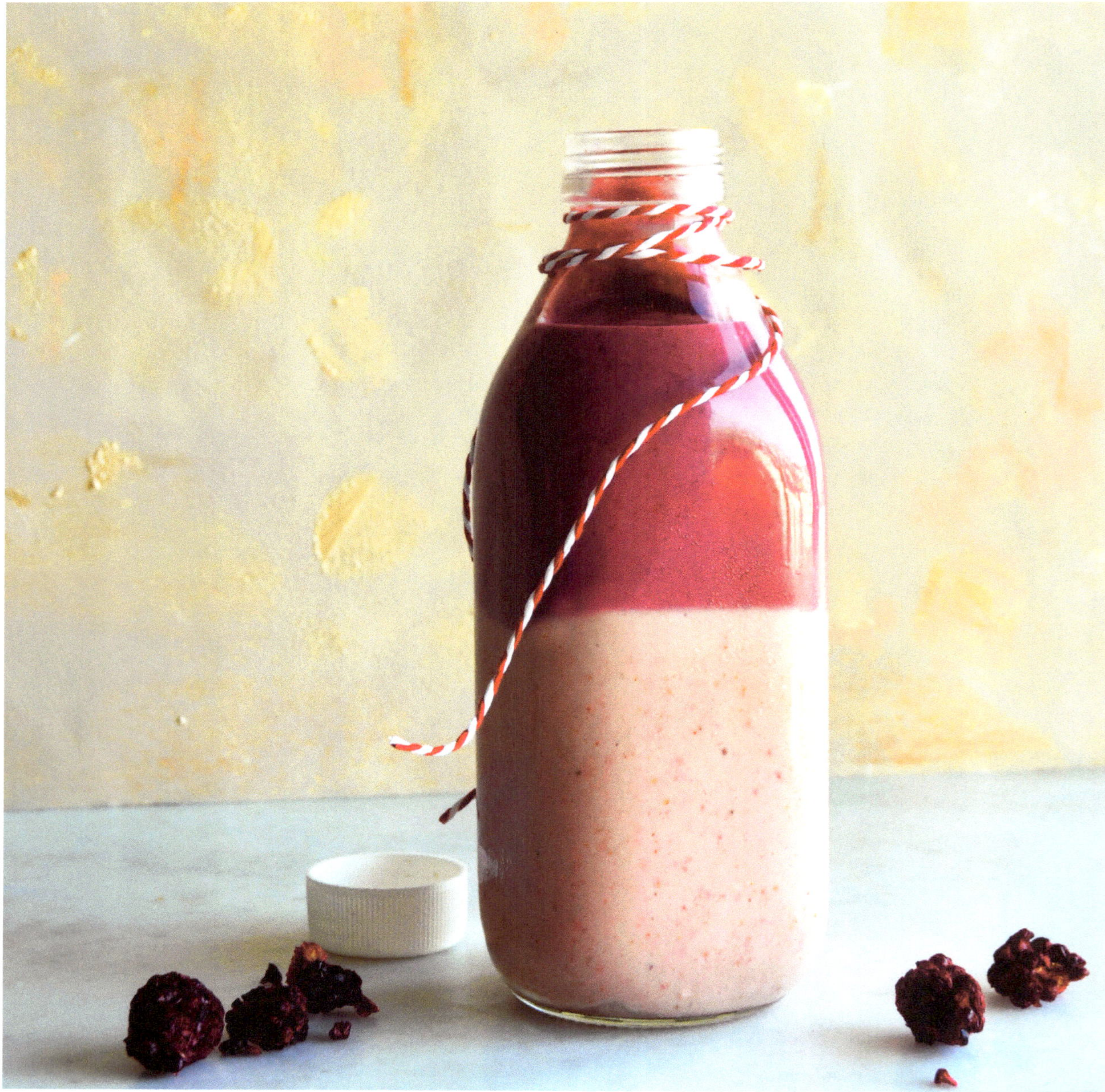

ROSA SMOOTHIE

Category - Pure-Raw
Preperation - 15 min + 20 min setting
Quantity - 2-3 person
Equipment - High speed blender
Storage - Up to 2 days in the fridge

Blackberry Layer Ingredients
200 g semi-frozen bananas
125 g semi-frozen blackberries
30 g soft medjool dates pitted
1 tsp carob powder
1 tbsp unroasted tahini
60 ml coconut milk

Strawberry Layer Ingredients
200 g semi-frozen bananas
100 g semi-frozen strawberries
12 g peeled fresh ginger
1/2 tsp maca powder
1 tbsp unroasted tahini
100 ml coconut milk

Instructions
1. To make strawberry layer, place all ingredients to a high speed blender. (we recommend Blendtec with wild-side jar for smoothies. It works great!) Blend on high speed for 25-30 seconds until you get smooth mixture. Then transfer mixture to a 600 ml bottle. Fill the half of the bottle with strawberry layer.
2. To make blackberry layer, place all ingredients listed to your Blendtec. Blend on high speed until smooth. Taste and adjust if you need. The consistency should be a thick in order to make two color smoothie in the bottle. But if it is too thick add some more coconut milk depending on your preference. Consistency may change due to juice inside the fruit or coconut milk you choose. Homemade coconut milk works well or unsweetened packaged one goes well too.
3. When it is done, pour the blackberry layer over the strawberry yogurt layer in the bottle. It is ready to drink!
Tip: To avoid mixing of two layers, first pour the first layer into the bottle using a funnel. Then wait for 15-20 minutes to cool in the fridge. Transfer the second layer on to it with the help of a funnel. Enjoy!

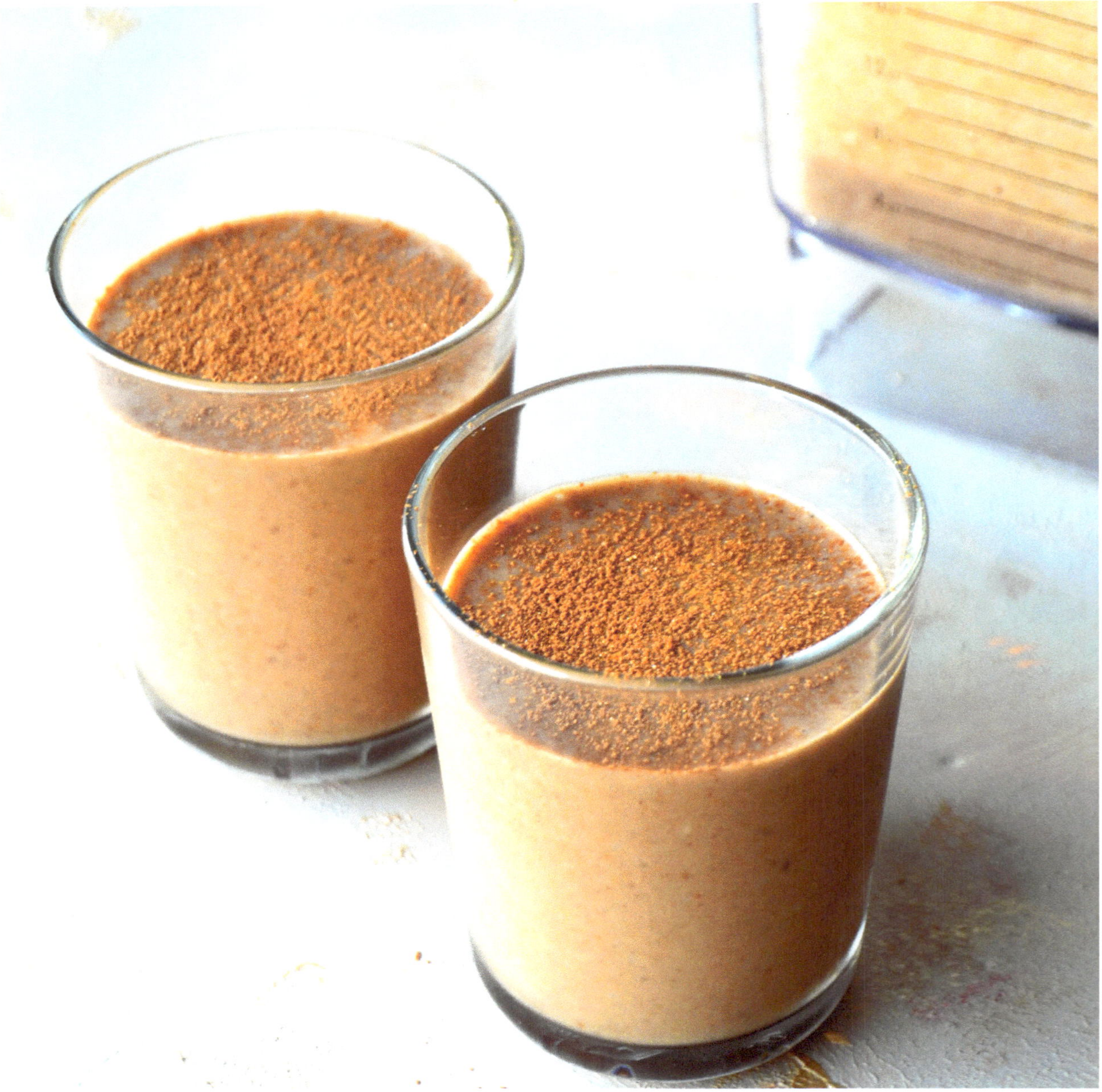

MOCHA SMOOTHIE

Category - Pure-Raw
Preperation - 6 minutes
Quantity - 2 person

Equipment - High speed blender
Personal note - The natural energy you need to power through your day!

Ingredients

230 ml fresh coconut water
1/2 cup young coconut meat
2 frozen bananas
1 tbsp raw cacao powder
1 tbsp almond butter
1 tsp maca powder
1/8 tsp vanilla
1/4 tsp pink himalayan salt

Instructions

1. Place fresh coconut water and coconut meat into your blender. Mix on high speed until smooth.
2. Add frozen bananas, almond butter, raw cacao powder, vanilla, maca and salt. Continue to blend until combined well.
3. Pour into glasses.
4. Dust some raw cacao powder and serve cold!

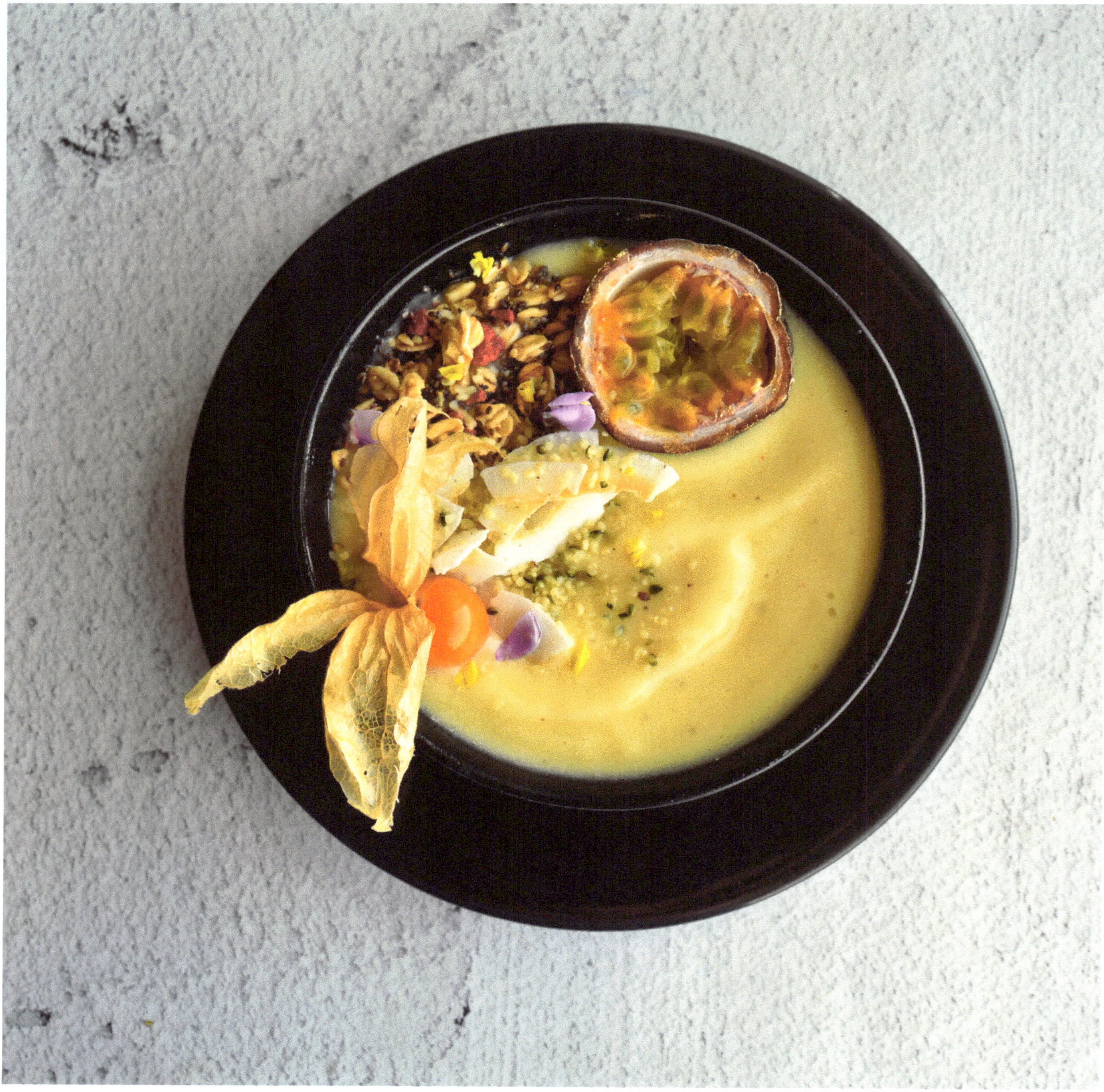

TROPICAL ISLAND SMOOTHIE

Category - Pure-Raw
Preperation - 15 minutes

Equipment - High speed blender
Quantity - 2 person

Ingredients

100 g semi-frozen bananas
200 g semi-frozen pineapple
50 g frozen physalis or mango
1 tbsp irish moss gel
5 cm fresh ginger
2.5 cm fresh turmeric
1 tbsp lime juice

Toppings

1 tbsp hemp hearts
2 tbsp oat or buckwheat granola (page 31)
1 tbsp coconut chips
1 physalis and passion fruit
Freeze dried berries
Bean blossom to decorate (optional)

Instructions

1. Add the banana, pineapple ginger, lime juice, turmeric, irish moss gel and physalis to your blender. Blend until smooth and creamy. Use the ice cream mode if you are using Blendtec or blend on your high speed option until smooth.
2. Top with hemp hearts, granola, freeze dried forest berries, coconut chips, passion fruit and physalis. Decorate with bean blossoms. Enjoy cold!

How to make irish moss gel?

Irish Moss is a seaweed sometimes considered healing to the digestive tract, maybe even a superfood, often used as a thickening agent. To make irish moss gel, wash 1 cup moss twice and soak it overnight, in the morning remove the sea moss from the water, and transfer it to a high-speed blender along with the clean water. Use 1 cup water to start and add more depending on the consistency you would like your gel. Blend until it is smooth, about 1-3 minutes. Transfer the irish moss into an airtight container/mason jar and refrigerate. The sea moss gel will thicken in the fridge after 2 hours.

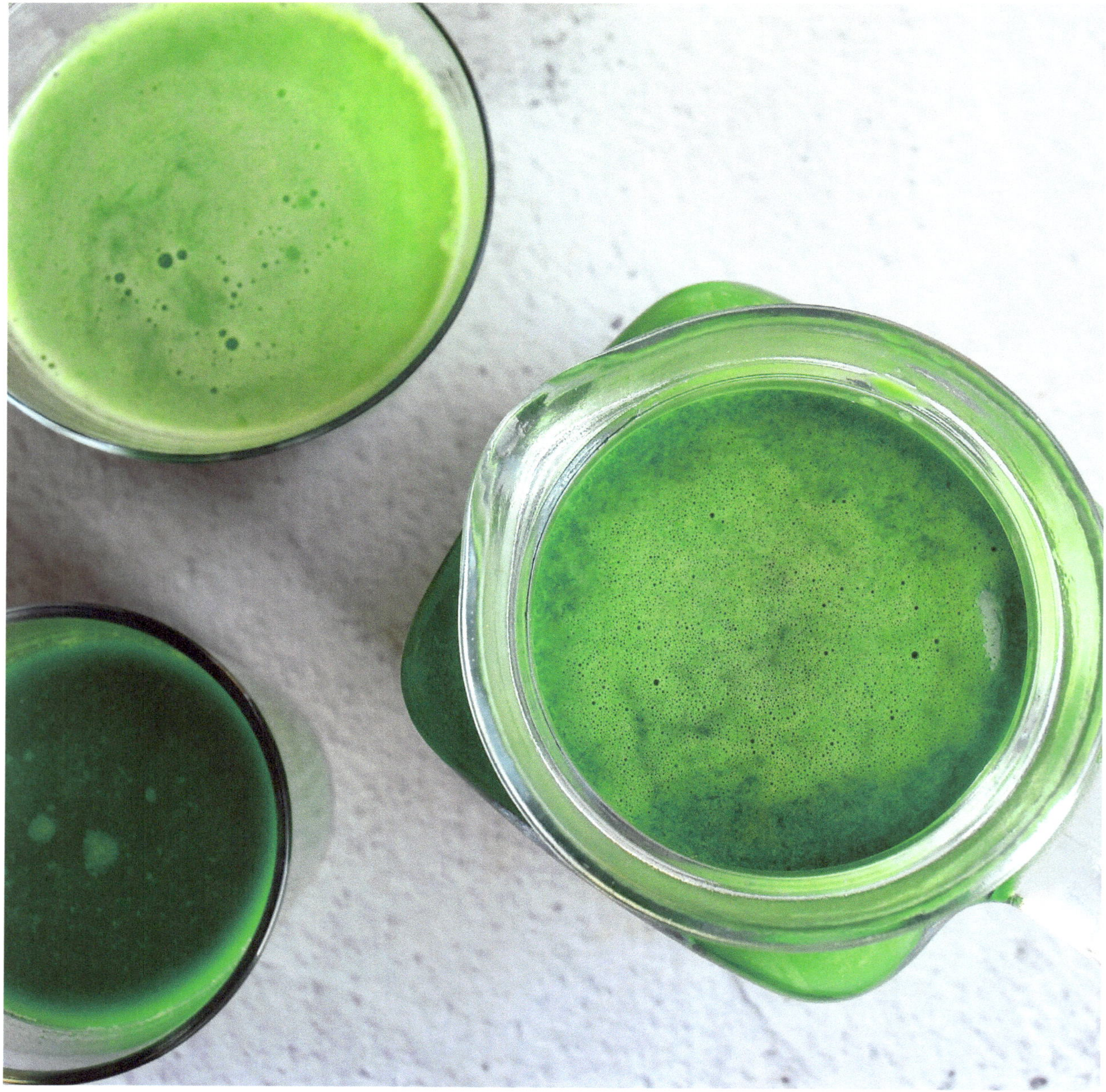

HEALING GREEN JUICE

The easiest way to enjoy the benefits of a green juice is to drink it as your breakfast. It is also a detoxifying agent, because it binds to heavy metals and toxins in your body. You will find that when you consume more dark green vegetables, you also experience an increase in your energy level. We like to use moisture-rich celery and cucumber as a base, then add kale for pungent green color. Apple adds a touch of sweetness, while fennel, ginger and lime add tangy flavor. Enjoy this balanced healing green juice.

Category - Pure raw
Time - 20 min
Equipment - Juicer
Quantity - 1 person

Ingredients
1 cup kale
10 cm fennel
5 celery stalks
2 large cucumber
3 green apples
1 lime
5 cm ginger

Instructions
1. Chop all vegetables into small pieces enough to fit easily down the chute.
2. Peel all citrus fruits as they can be difficult for the machine to process, which inhibits them from being fully juiced.
3. Run all ingredients through the juicer, using your tamper as needed.
4. Strain your juice to get a better texture, if you prefer.
5. Pour in to a clean bottle or glass.
6. Enjoy juice fresh or within 24 hours for best flavor. You can also keep it in a jar or sealed container in the fridge for up to 48 hours depending on your juicer.

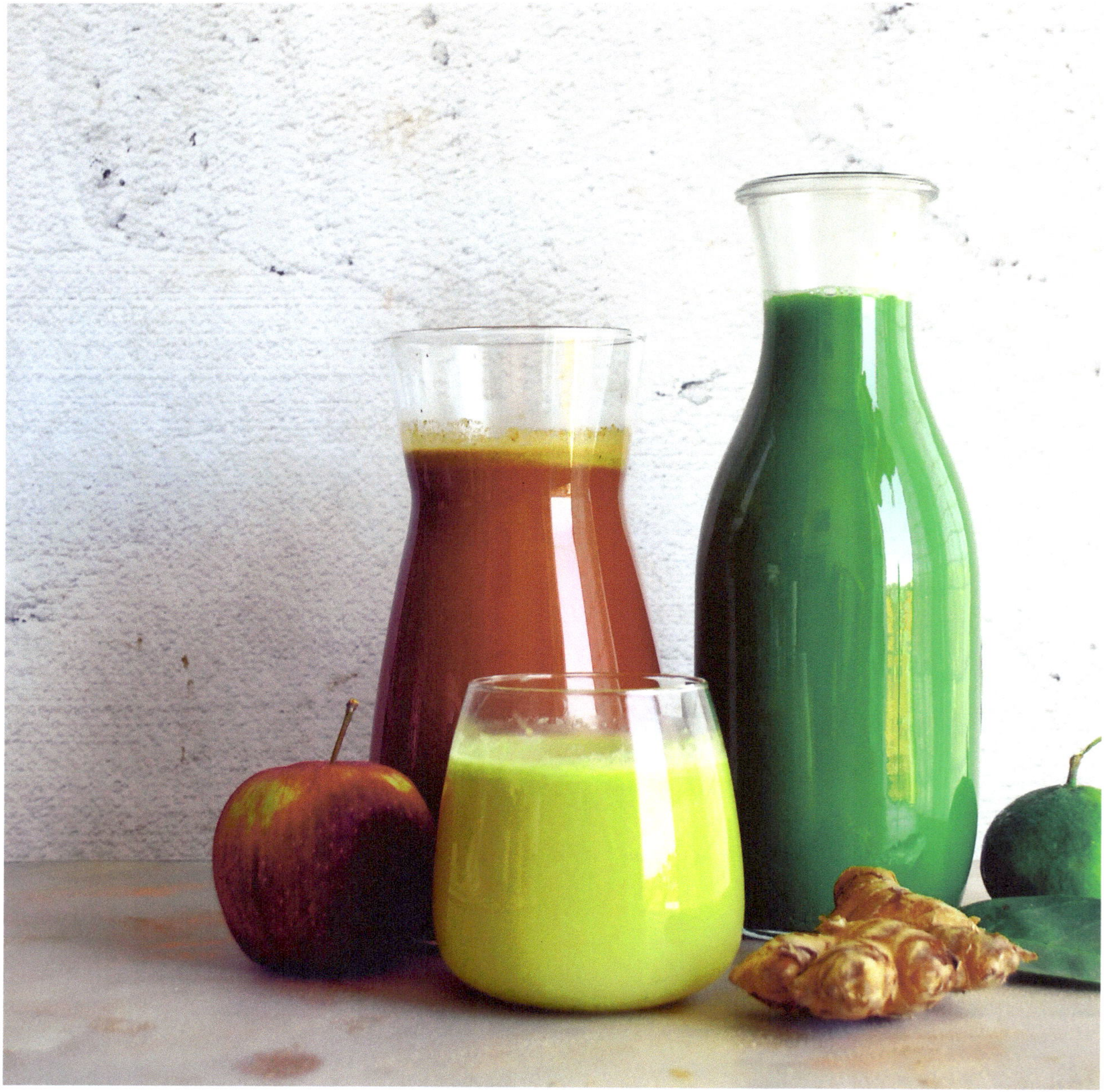

CANDY JUICE

This juice recipe will provide you with the natural glucose and mineral salts your body needs to heal and thrive. Apples are a truly healing food. They are anti-inflammatory because they starve viruses. This fruit helps cleanse and purify the organs, improve circulation in your lymphatic system, repair damaged skin, and regulate blood sugar.

Apples are also hydrating on a deep, cellular level. They provide precious trace minerals such as manganese and molybdenum, as well as electrolytes and critical mineral salts that help the body rehydrate after exercise or stress of any kind. And the addition of cinnamon takes this juice to a new level of deliciousness.

Ingredients

4 red apples
5 celery stalks
5 cm ginger
1 tsp cinnamon

Instructions

In a juicer, juice the apples, celery, and ginger. Stir in the cinnamon and serve.

SUNSHINE JUICE

Ingredients

1 golden apple
5 tangerines
1 whole lemon
5 cm ginger

Instructions

1. Run all the ingredients through the juicer.
2. Drink the juice immediately on an empty stomach for best results.

contemporary entrées

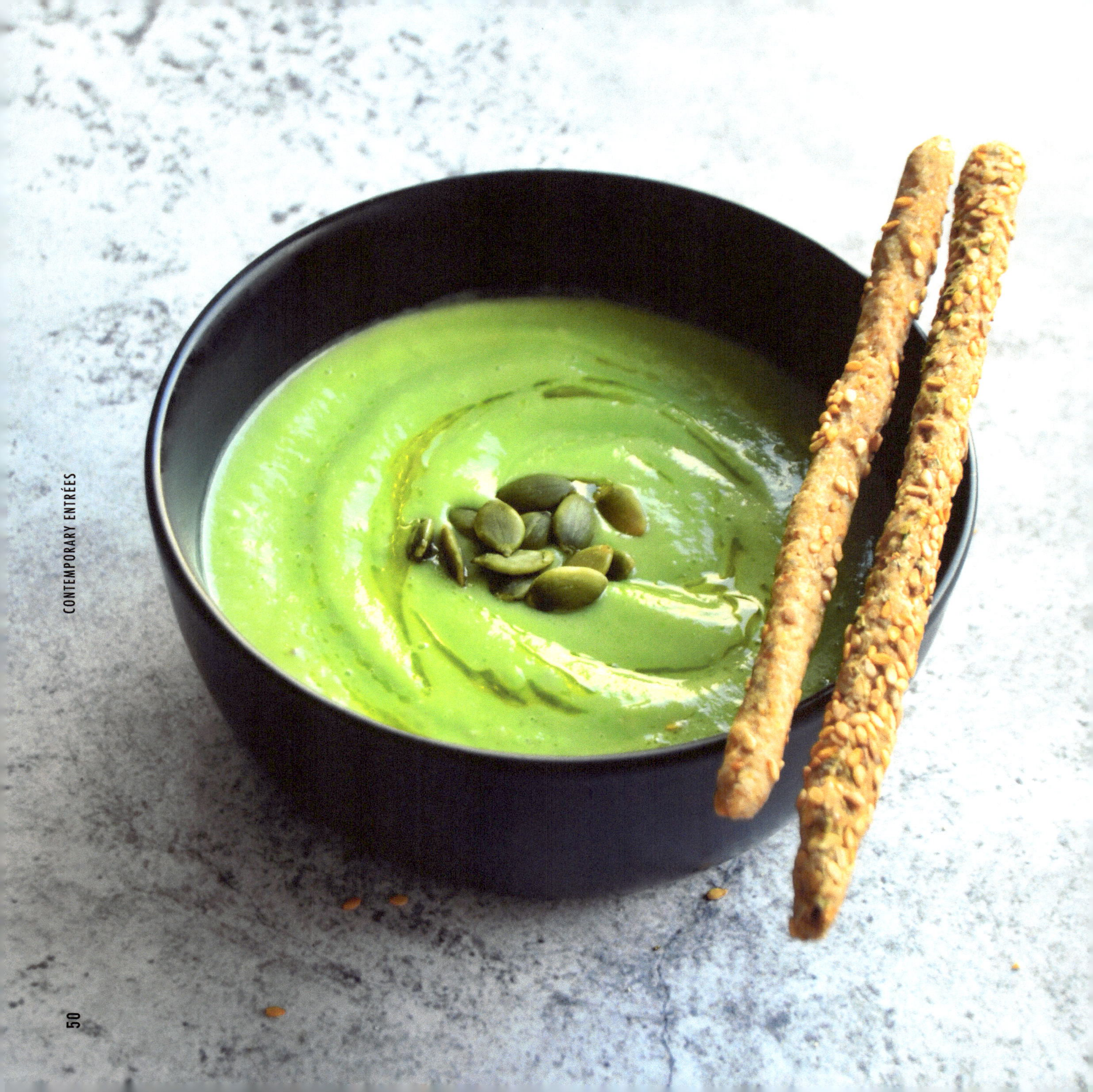

GINGER BROCCOLI SOUP

Category - Sous Vide-Raw
Time - 15 min prep + 30 min sous vide
Quantity - 2 person

Equipment - Sous vide, blender

Why sous vide? - Broccoli can be easily overcooked using traditional methods such as boiling or roasting. It will turn brown and tastes terrible. Sous vide method makes the best broccoli with a perfect texture by controlling the temperature precisely.

Ingredients

450 g broccoli
1 medium onion
15 g ginger peeled
3 cups water
1 tsp salt
Pepper to taste
1/2 lemon juice
1 ripe hass type avocado
1 tbsp olive oil

Instructions

1. After cleaning your broccoli, break the crown apart into big florets and then slice them into bite-sized pieces. Peel the stems and cut it into thin slices.
2. Peel your onion and cut into two.
3. Place broccoli pieces and onion in a vacuum bag or in a zip-top bag and seal.
4. Drizzle with olive oil, and season with salt and pepper, add peeled ginger in the bag.
5. Cook at 42° C for 30 minutes for a crispier texture with a vibrant green color. Cook at 46 °C for 40-45 minutes if you like more tender broccoli, but the color turns brownish.
6. Once cooked, transfer broccoli and ginger to a blender. Add the water and peeled de-seeded avocado. Blend until silky smooth. Add more water if you need.
7. Squeeze lemon juice right before serving for a refreshing taste.

ginger broccoli soup continued

Tips for sous vide cooking: To prevent the vacuum-sealed bags from floating, you can use sous vide weights and place them in the bag with your broccoli to weigh down the bag. Alternatively, use heavy kitchen items such as metal tongs and heavy bowls to keep it fully submerged

BUCKWHEAT GRISSINI

Category - Dehydrated-Raw
Time - 20 min prep + 8 hrs dehydration

Equipment - food processor, dehydrator, oil brush
Quantity - 20 sticks

Ingredients

1 cup buckwheat
2 tbsp coconut sugar
1 tbsp psyllium powder
1/2 cup shredded pumpkin
1 large zucchini peeled
1 tbsp chopped green olives
Sesame seeds to sprinkle
1 tbsp olive oil

Instructions

1.Wash, rinse and drain the buckwheat. Allow to sprout until you see little tails. Place the buckwheat on teflex-lined sheets in a dehydrator set to 46° C and dehydrate for 6-8 hours or until completely dried.
2. Grind sprouted dehydrated buckwheats into a fine meal in a food processor.

3. Add the rest of the ingredients. Process till you have a sticky dough. If your dough is too dry, add more water until it's still thick, but pliable.

4. Take the dough out of your food processor and transfer to a lightly almond floured surface.

5. Using your hands, knead it for about 2-3 minutes. Divide your dough into 20 equal pieces.

6. Take each piece and stretch with your fingers to form long sticks.

7. Place the sticks on dehydrator sheets lined silicon paper, leaving some space in between them as they will bake slightly while in the dehydrator.

8. Using an oil brush, gently apply some olive oil over the top of the breadsticks then sprinkle some sea salt and sesame seeds on top.

9. Bake at 46° C for 6-8 hours.

10. After 8 hours you will need to remove the silicon paper and flip them on the other side, continue to bake for 2-3 hours or until crispy enough. Serve with your soup.

Notes: pumpkin can be replaced with carrot or root veggies like kohlrabi, swede etc.

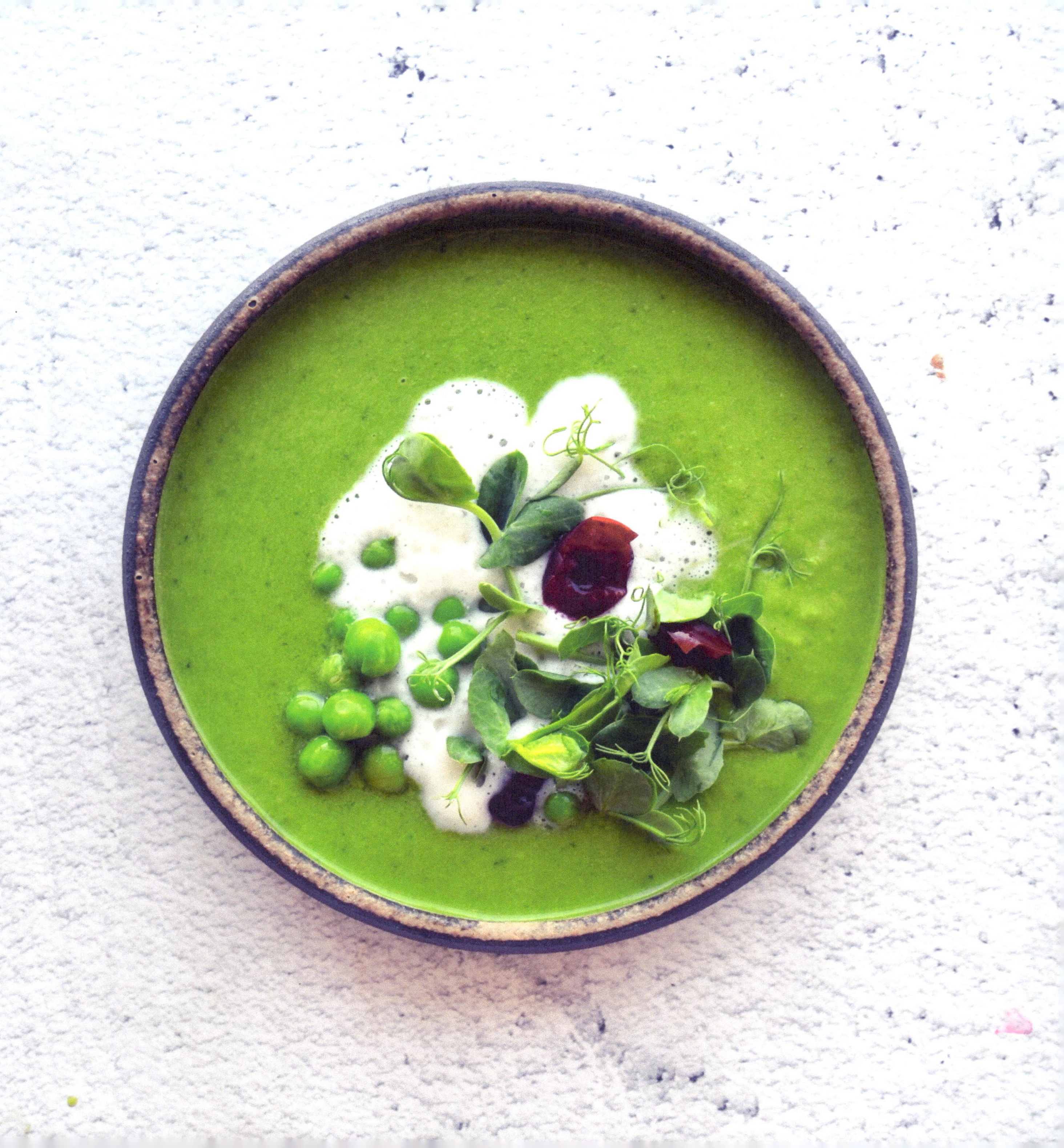

SPRING SOUP WITH COCONUT FOAM

Category - Dehydrated-Raw

Time - 20 min prep + 8 hrs dehydration

Quantity - 2 person

Equipment - Food processor, dehydrator

Personal note - Spring feelings

Ingredients

1 small onion

2 cups water

1/2 bunch swiss chard or spinach

1/2 cup fresh baby green peas

70 g fresh baby asparagus

2 large zucchinis

1 tbsp olive oil

Salt and chili to taste

Coconut foam

1/2 cup coconut cream

1/2 cup coconut milk

1 tsp sunflower lecithin or soy lecithin

4 tbsp lemon juice

1/2 tsp salt

Cherries and pea sprouts to decorate

Instructions

1. Wash and dry swiss chard, asparagus and peas. Add 1/2 tbsp olive oil, massage well.
2. Peel your zucchini and onion, thinly slice. Add 1/2 tbsp olive oil, massage.
3. On a dehydrator tray with silicon paper, place swiss chard leaves.
4. On the second dehydrator tray with silicon sheet, place asparagus thinly sliced asparagus, onion, garlic and zucchini. Sprinkle some salt.
5. On the third dehydrator tray, place the rest of the asparagus, zucchini, onions with some distance between so that they do not stick together.
6. Dehydrate at 42° C for 2-3 hours or until semi-dehydrated. We want them soft not crispy so check regularly during the dehydration process.
7. Once done, transfer all dehydrated veggies to your food processor. Add 2 cups water and blend until smooth. Then transfer to a sieve, strain the soup. Remove the pulp.
8. In a food processor, blend coconut cream, coconut milk and lecithin until you get foam. This process can take anywhere from 60 seconds up to a few minutes. Let the foam stabilize for a minute and then you can use it.
9. Serve soup with coconut foam, cherries, fresh baby peas and pea sprouts.

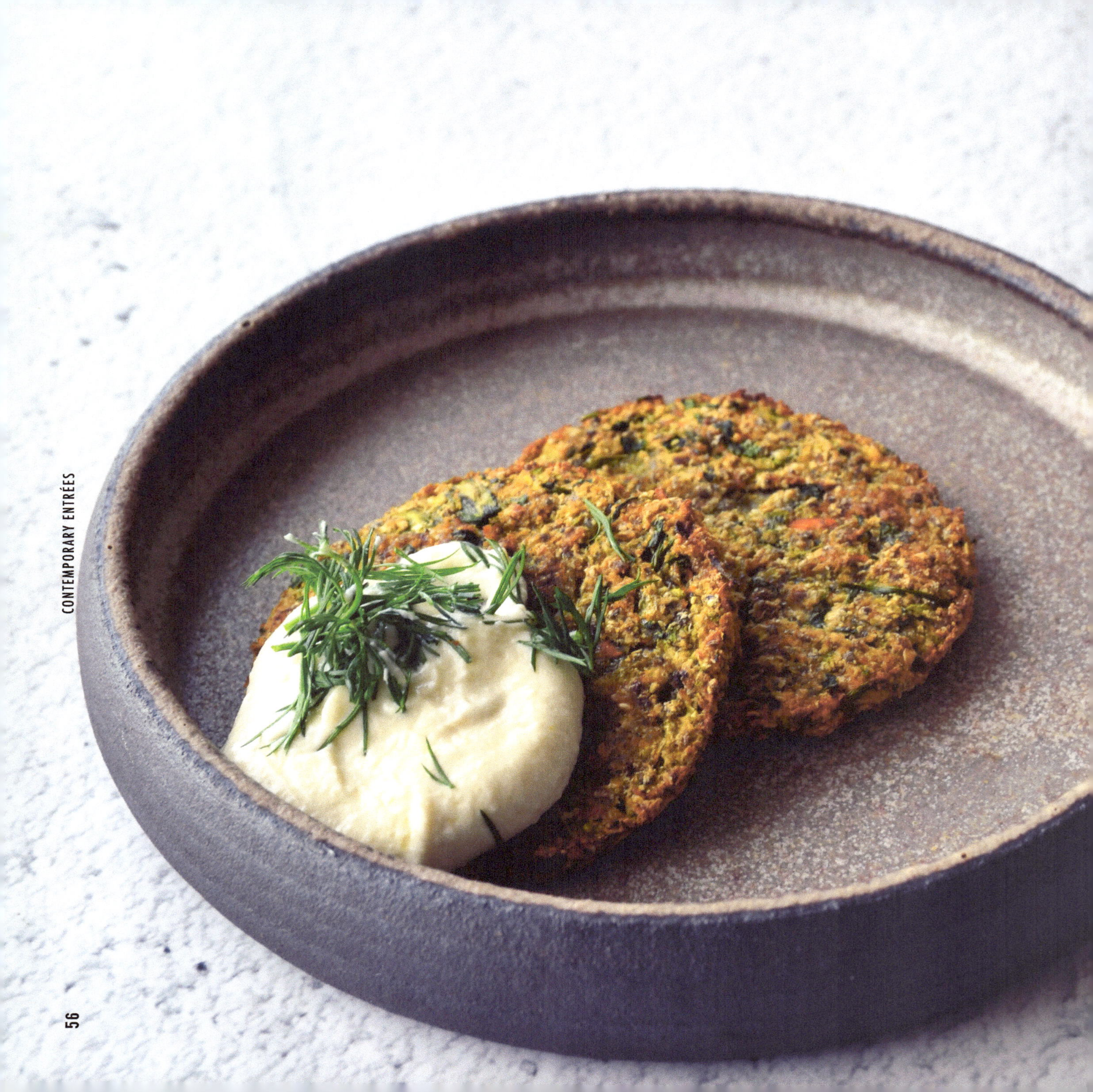

ZUCCHINI MÜCVER WITH YOGURT

Category - Pure-Raw +Dehydrated-Raw
Time - 25 min prep + 7 hrs dehydration

Equipment - Food processor, blender, spatula, dehydrator
Quantity - 3-4 person

Zucchini mücver

3 zucchinis (450g) shredded
1 carrot (32g) shredded
3 tbsp chia seeds
1 tbsp psyllium husk powder
3 tbsp sprouted oat flour
1 tsp baking powder
1 tsp minced garlic
1/4 cup chopped parsley
2-3 springs green onion
1 tsp pink himalayan salt
1/4 tsp black pepper and chili

Not-fermented cashew yogurt

120 g raw cashews soaked (or young coconut meat or macadamias)
6 tbsp fresh lemon juice
5 tbsp filtered water
1 tbsp olive oil
2 tsp minced garlic
1/4 tsp black pepper
1/4 tsp pink himalayan salt

Instructions

1. **To make mücver**, peel and shred your veggies, squeeze out the excess water. Transfer excess water in a bowl. Add the chia seeds in this water, let it sit for 5 min until chia absorbs the water.
2. Add the veggies, chia mixture and rest of the ingredients to the food processor, blend until get dough form. It may seem too dry at first, but keep stirring, it will start to stick.
3. Divide the dough into 4 pieces, form balls, then flatten out into little patties about 1.3 cm thick.
4. Place onto parchment paper and chill in the fridge for 30 minutes to firm up some.
5. Once the time is almost up, dehydrate patties at 42° C for 7-8 hours in the dehydrator. Then carefully flip them over with a spatula, continue to dehydrate for 3-4 hours.
6. **To make yogurt,** place all the yogurt ingredients to the blender. Blend until silky smooth.
7. Keep in the fridge for 1 hour before serving. The sauce will thicken the longer it sits.
8. Serve with yogurt and chopped fresh dill.

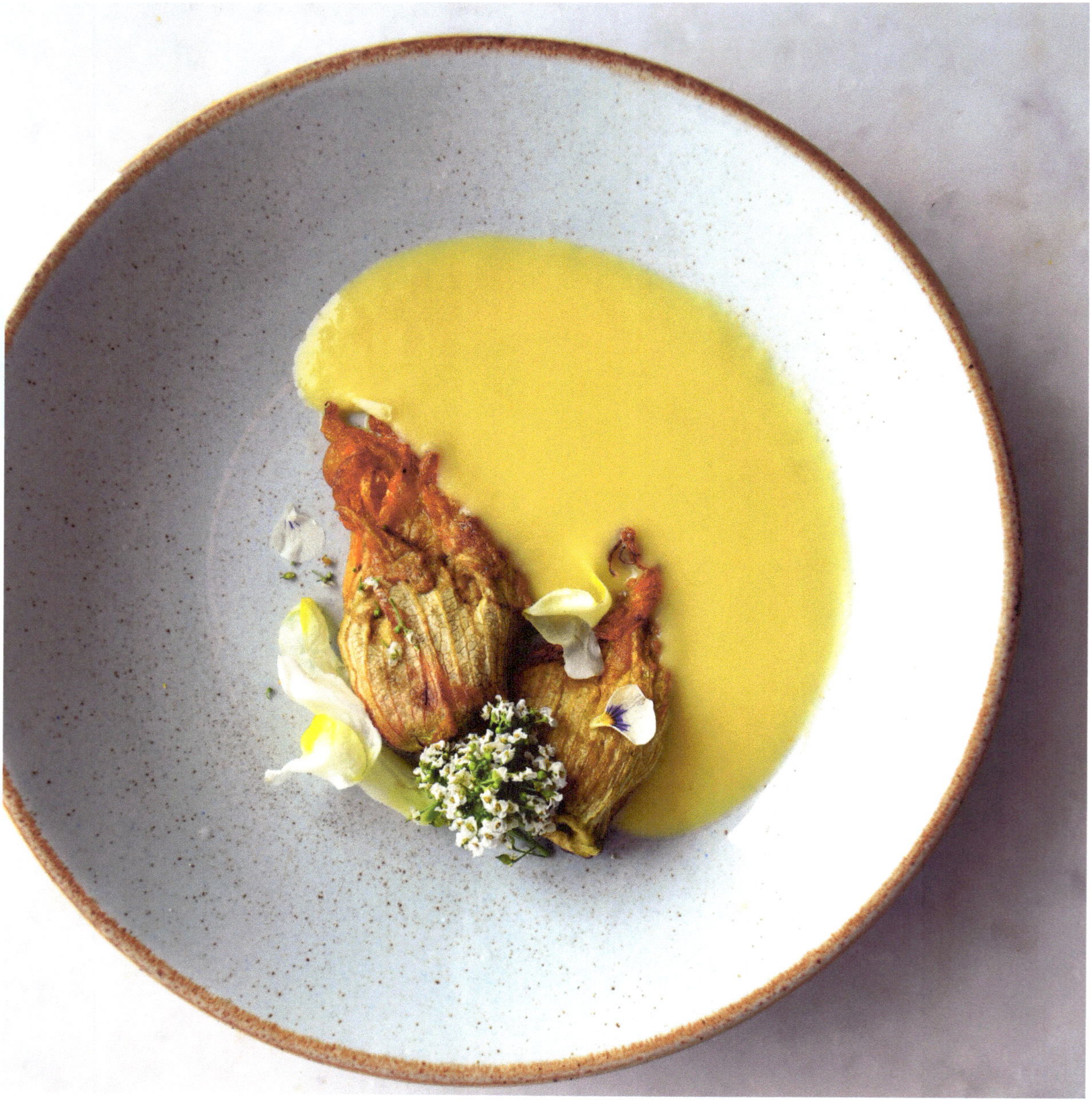

STUFFED ZUCCHINI BLOSSOMS AND GINGER BISQUE

Category - Dehydrated-Raw

Time - 20 min prep + 6 hrs dehydration

Equipment - Blender, dehydrator

Quantity- 3-4 person

Ingredients

10-12 zucchini blossoms

Ginger Bisque

1 large onion

1 large carrot

1 tbsp minced ginger

1 tbsp grated orange peel

2 cups water

1 tbsp olive oil

Filling cream with basil

80 g sunflower seeds

1 tbsp nutritional yeast

1 tsp dijon mustard or 3 tbsp lemon juice

6-7 tbsp water to blend

1 tbsp garlic minced

1 tsp salt or miso

1 tsp blackpepper

2 tbsp chopped fresh basil

To make filling with basil

1. Soak sunflower seeds for 1 hour then rinse and dry. Place into a high speed blender, add the rest of the ingredients. Blend well until smooth.

To make ginger bisque

1. Thinly slice onion and carrot, dehydrate for 4-5 hours until semi-dehydrated.
2. Transfer them to a high speed food processor, add the rest of the ingredients. Blend until smooth. Using a sieve, strain the mixture, remove the pulp.
3. Transfer half of the mixture of the bisque into a small sauce server to serve later. Set aside other half in a large bowl. We will use it as a batter.

Assembly

1. Wash and dry your zucchini blossoms. Carefully open each blossom and fill about 2 tsp filling cream. Gently twist end of blossom to enclose filling.
2. Dip zucchini blossoms in ginger bisque batter. Coat well.
3. Place them onto a dehydrator tray with silicon sheets. Dehydrate at 42° C for 4-5 hours or until completely dried. Then place into your plate.
4. Using a sauce server, pour ginger bisque around the zucchini blossom. Decorate with dragon snaps, alyssum and white viola if desired.

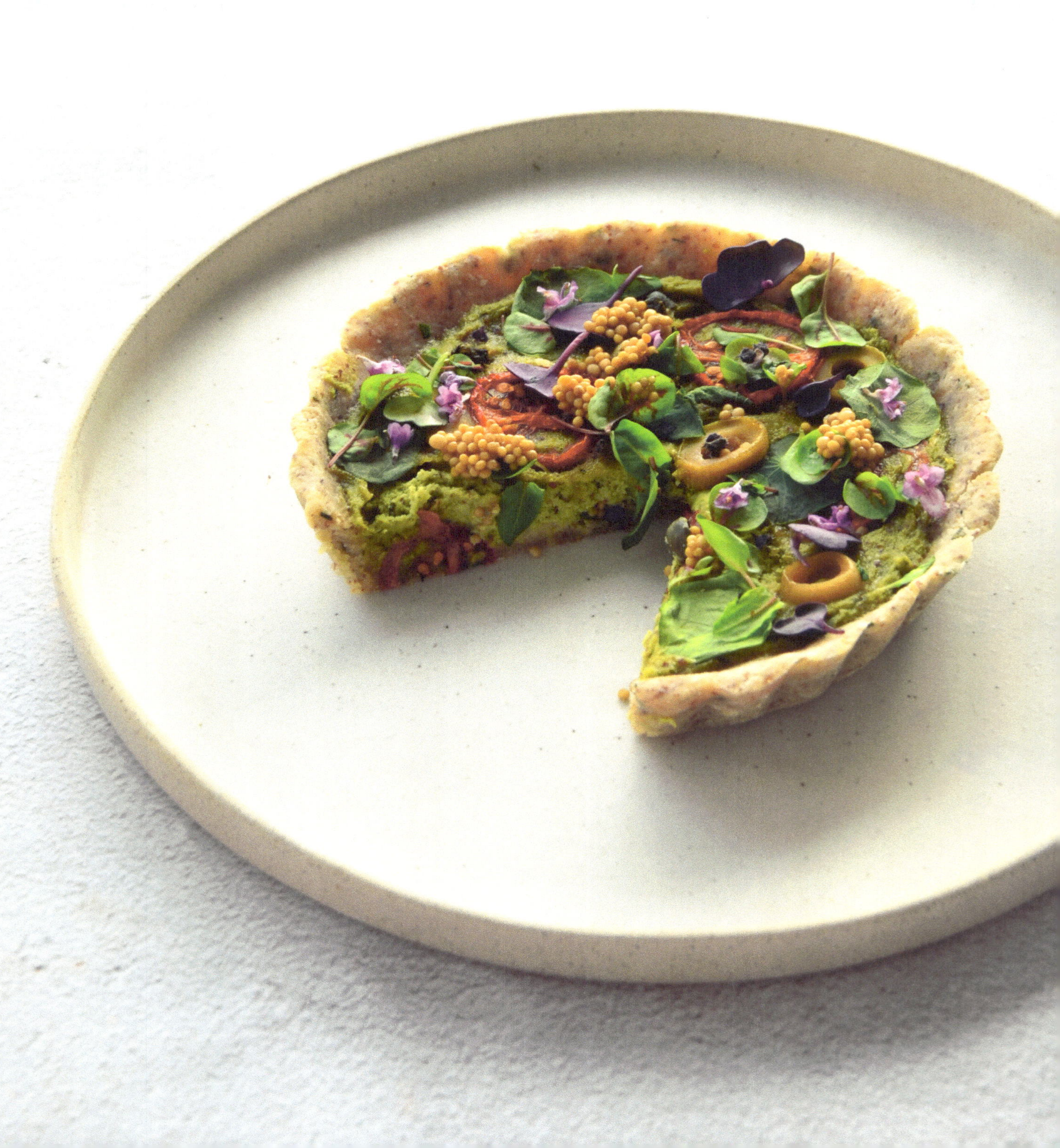

ALMOND QUICHE WITH SPIRULINA HORSERADISH CREAM

Category - Dehydrated-Raw
Time - 15 min prep + 4 hrs dehydration
Quantity - 4 x 7cm tart

Equipment - Food processor, dehydrator, 7cm tart tin

Quiche crust ingredients

2 cups soaked almonds
1 tbsp almond oil
4 tbsp ground flaxseed
4 tbsp nutritional yeast
3 tbsp freshly chopped rosemary
1/2 tsp salt
1 tbsp lemon juice
1 tsp garlic powder
1/2 cup water

Instructions

1. Place almonds, flaxseed, nutritional yeast, salt, garlic and rosemary in a food processor. Pulse to combine.
2. Add the water, almond oil and lemon juice. Process for a minute or two, stopping to scrape the bowl down. Add more water as needed, until the mixture is easily spreadable (not liquidly, but not at all pasty, either).
3. Press mixture into a non-stick quiche pan with removable bottom.
4. Dehydrate at 46°C for 1 hour. Decrease heat to 36°C and continue to dehydrate about 3 hours or until completely dried.

almond quiche continued

Horseradish cream ingredients

1 cup activated almonds

1 tbsp grated fresh horseradish

1 cup almond milk

2 tbsp nutritional yeast

1 tsp miso

1 tbsp lemon juice

1 shallot chopped

1 tbsp olive oil

1 tsp spirulina

Toppings

Sliced cherry tomatoes

Sliced green olives

Mustard caviar

Microgreens

Fresh basil

Preferred greens

To make horseradish cream

1. Place soaked and strained almonds into your blender, add almond milk. Blend until you get a smooth cream. You may need to add more almond milk to achieve the desired consistency. It should be a thick pourable cream, not too liquid, not too thick.
2. Add grated horseradish, nutritional yeast, miso, lemon juice, chopped shallot, olive oil and spirulina. Continue to blend until smooth.
3. Pour mixture over the quiche crusts.
4. Slice tomatoes and green olives thinly, add to your quiche.
5. Dehydrate at 42° C for 5-6 hours or until completely dried.
6. Serve with mustard caviar, fresh greens and microgreens.

SOFT CAULIFLOWER BREAD

Category - Dehydrated-Raw
Time - 20 min prep + 8 hrs dehydration

Equipment - Food processor, dehydrator
Quantity- 6 buns

Bread ingredients

450 g cauliflower riced
190 g zucchini peeled
3 tbsp nutritional yeast
2 tbsp chia seeds
1/2 cup psyllium husk
1 tsp salt
1/4 cup water

Avocado mayo

2/3 cup mashed ripe avocados
1 tbsp lemon juice
2 tsp apple cider vinegar
3/4 tsp onion powder
1 tsp minced garlic
1/4 tsp salt
1/4 cup water

Toppings

Halved cherry tomatoes
Capers
Mustard caviar
Microgreens

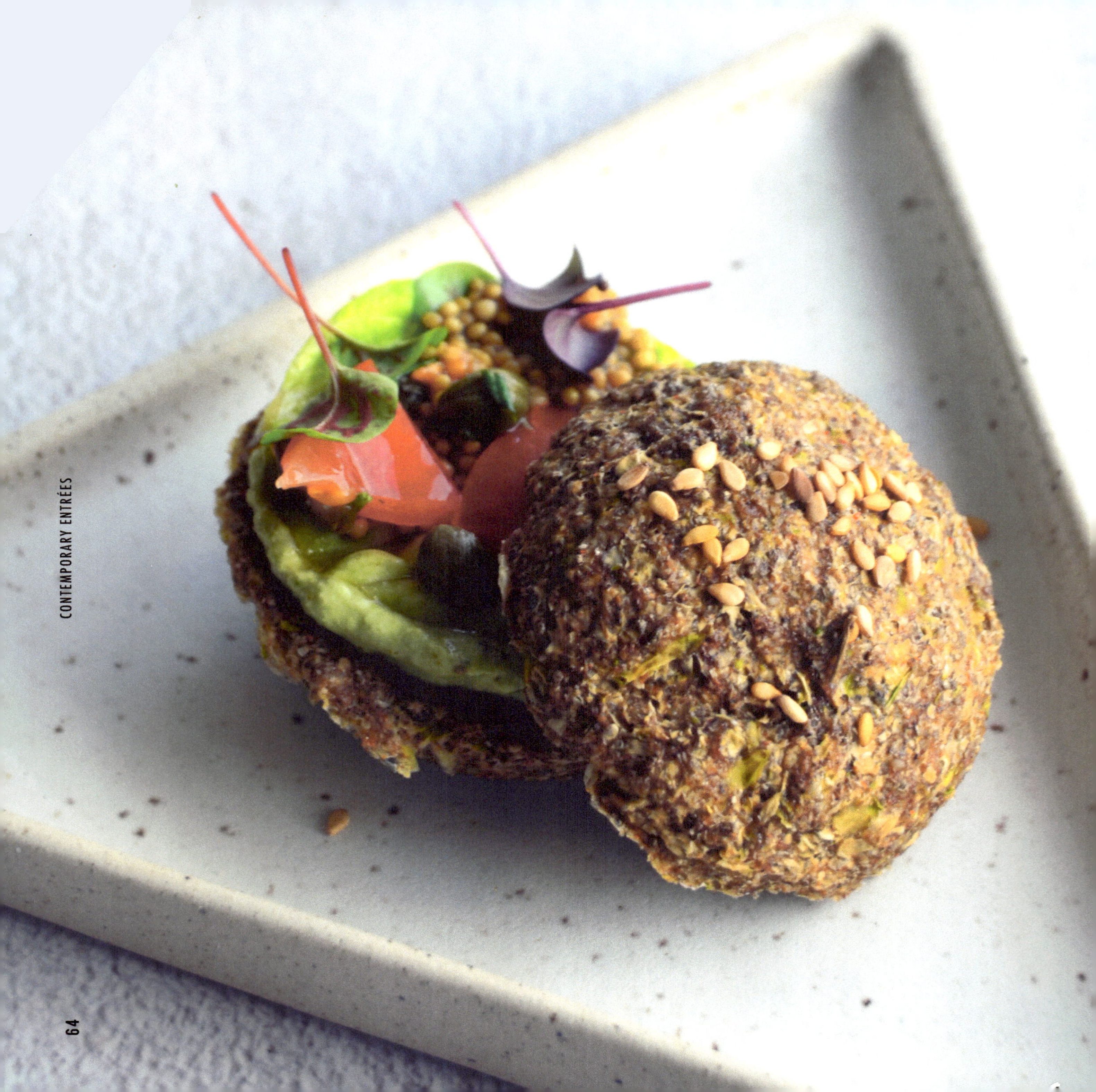

Instructions

1. Peel, wash and cut your zucchini. Transfer to the food processor.
2. Wash and chop your cauliflower and add in your food processor, then pulse until completely broken down. (You can also replace cauliflower with zucchini or kohlrabi if you prefer.)
3. In a coffee grinder, grind the chia seeds, then add to your food processor. (Do not skip chia seeds, adding both chia seeds and psyllium husk to dough recipes makes it fluffy and moist.)
4. Add the rest of the ingredients. Then process until fully combined.
5. Form mixture into bread balls on your dehydrator sheets (you will get around 8 balls), you can use a silicon mould to make this.
6. Dehydrate for 6 hours for a soft bread, for a crispy one, dehydrate for about 8 hrs. You can also flip the slices half-way through.
7. Once done, remove from the dehydrator.
8. In a small bowl, combine halved cherry tomatoes, capers and olive oil.
9. In blendtec twister jar, combine all ingredients until smooth. Add more water if a thinner mayo spread is desired. If you want a spicy mayo, feel free to add a dash of cayenne.
10. Spread mayo onto the bread. Top your bread tomatoes and capers. Enjoy.

Storage: the bread can be kept in the fridge up to 4-5 days. Redehydrate at 42° C for 35-40 minutes or so before eating.

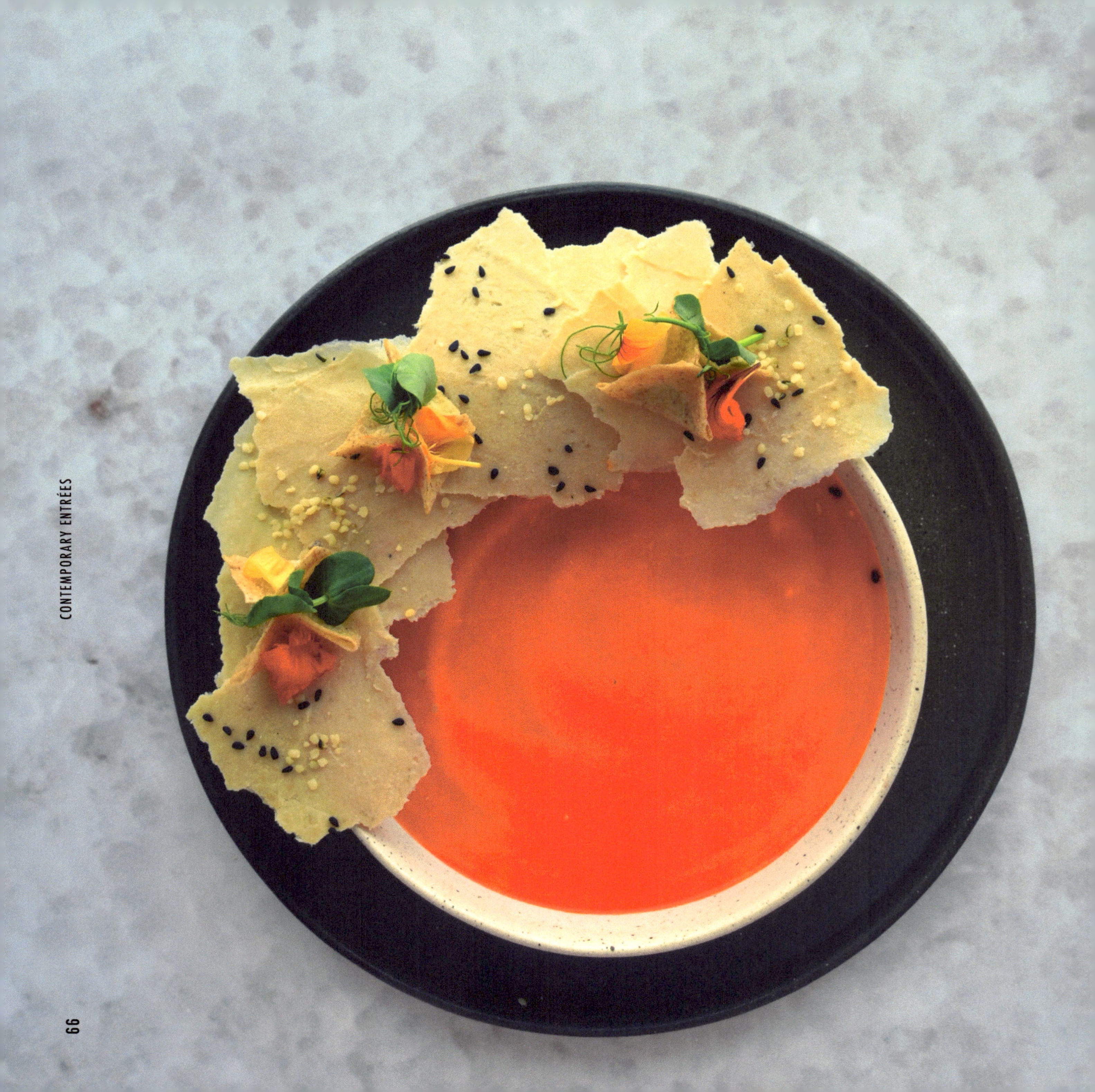

RED BELL PEPPER SOUP WITH BRIDAL TUILE & KOHLRABI MANTI

Category - Dehydrated- Raw
Preperation - 45 min + 24 hrs dehydration
Quantity - 2 person

Equipment - High speed blender, dehydrator, chef tweezer, spatula
Personal note - Like a fine dining!

Soup ingredients

3 cups red bell pepper
200 g heirloom tomatoes
2 cups water
2 tbsp olive oil
1/2 tsp salt
1/4 tsp chili pepper

To make soup

1. Cut red bell peppers and tomatoes into 3mm slices or in half – remember, thicker slices will take longer to dry out.
2.Brush some olive oil and dehydrate at 46° C until for about 8 hours maximum, until they slightly take on a leathery texture but still pliable. They also can be cooked sous vide if you prefer.
3. Once tomatoes and peppers are cooked, place them into your blender. Add the water, chili and salt. Blend until smooth. Taste and adjust the seasonings.

red bell pepper soup continued

Bridal tuile ingredients

1 + 1/2 cup pine nuts

1/2 cup lemon juice

2-3 tbsp water as needed

1 tsp salt

1 tbsp black sesame

1 tbsp hemp hearts

To make the tuiles

1. Place all ingredients into a high speed blender. Blend until silky smooth.
2. Spread the mixture over the dehydrator tray lined silicon sheet, as thin as possible.
3. Sprinkle black sesame and hemp hearts.

Dehydrate at 42° C for about 8-12 hours or overnight until completely dried and crispy.

Mantı dough ingredients

190 g kohlrabi

1 tbsp sesame oil

2 tbsp psyllium husk powder

2 tbsp water

A pinch of salt

Mantı Filling

Ricotta (page 71)

To make mantı

1. Peel your kohlrabi, cut into small pieces.
2. Add the kohlrabi, sesame oil and water to your blender.
3. Blend well until you get smooth puree.
4. Add the psyllium husk powder. Blend again.
5. Spread mixture over the dehydrator sheets.
6. Dehydrate at 42° C for about 6 hours -until completely dried.
7. When done, cut the dough into squares.
8. Fill them with almond ricotta (recipe page 71)
9. Pinch the opposite corners to form a little a little pouch and press the seams together to seal firmly.

Assembly

1. Break the tuiles randomly. Place the edges of the tuile overlapping so that they stand on the side of your soup bowl (as seen on page 66).
2. Put manti pieces on the top of the bridal tuiles.
3. Place yellow and red nasturtium flower leaves with the help of a chef tweezer in 2 of the 4 slots of the manti. Put pea sprouts in the third slot, leaving fourth slot empty.
4. Pour the red bell pepper soup into your bowl. Serve immediately!

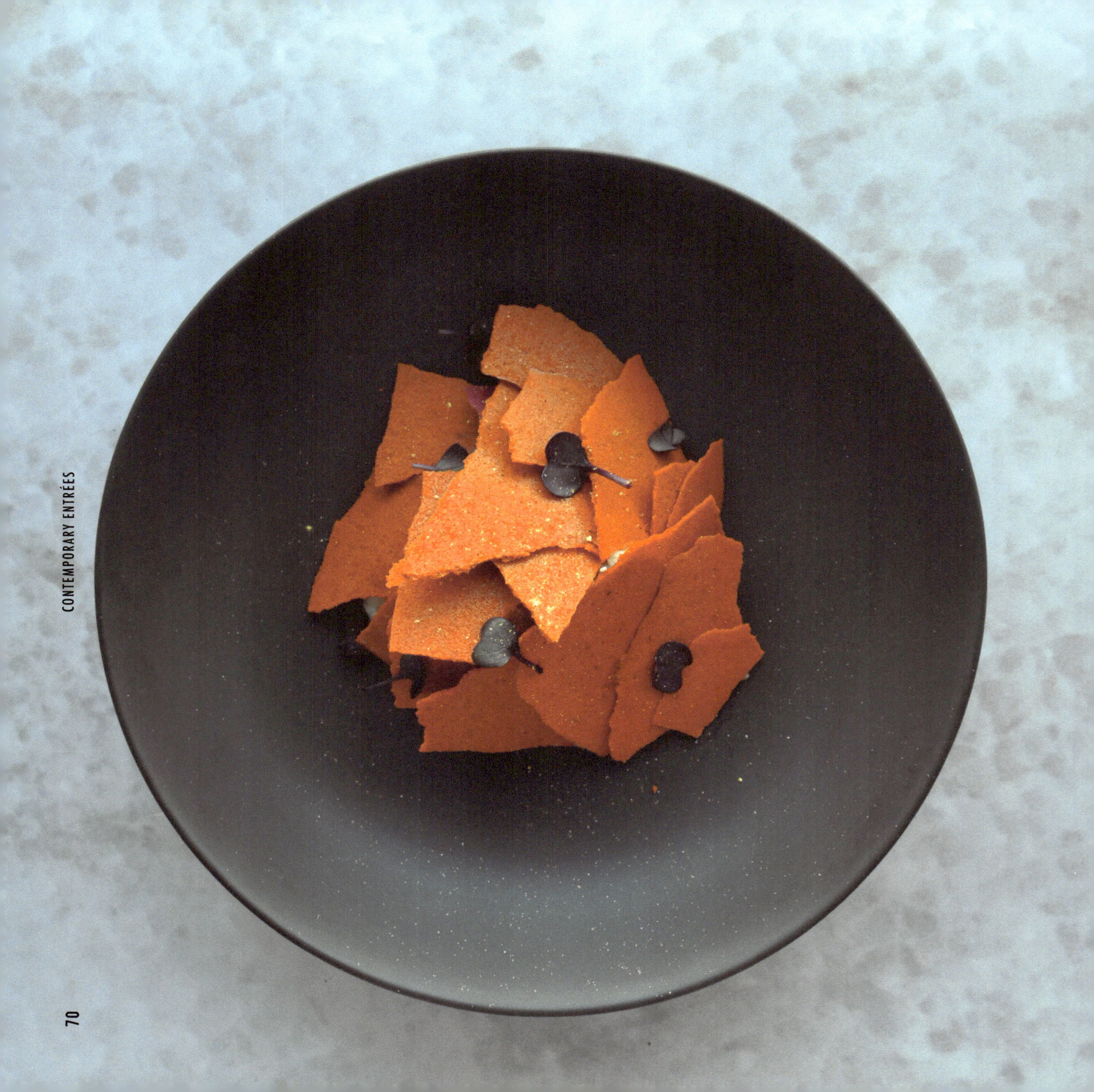

ALMOND RICOTTA WITH ORANGE AND TOMATO STROKES

Category - Dehydrated- Raw
Preperation - 45 min + 24 hrs dehydration
Quantity - 4-6 person

Equipment - High speed blender, spatula, dehydrator
Personal note - Like a fine dining!

Almond ricotta ingredients

2 cups blanched almonds
2 tbsp lemon juice
1/4 tsp garlic powder
1 cup water
2 tbsp fresh rosemary chopped
2 tbsp gluten free nutritional yeast

To make almond ricotta

1. Add all ricotta ingredients with the lesser amount of water to a high-speed blender and blend until smooth and creamy, scraping down sides as needed .
2. Add a bit more water a little at a time if the mixture is having a hard time blending until smooth.
3. Taste and adjust flavor as needed, adding more salt for overall flavor, nutritional yeast for cheesiness, and lemon juice for acidity. For even more flavor, you can add in fresh rosemary, chives or dill.
4. Wrap it, form in a ball, can be kept in the refrigerator up to 5 days.

Orange and tomato strokes ingredients

1 cup pine nuts (or sunflower seeds)
1 tbsp apple cider vinegar
3-4 tbsp lemon juice
2 pieces sundried tomatoes soaked
2 fresh cherry tomatoes
1 tsp freeze dried orange powder
1 tsp paprika powder
1 tsp salt
1/2 cup water

Other components

Red cabbage microgreens
Edible gold powder

To make orange and tomato strokes

1. Soak the pine nuts or sunflower seeds for 30 minutes. Rinse well and drain.
2. Add all ingredients into a blender and blend until it becomes a smooth cheese sauce.
3. Line a dehydrator tray with a silicon sheet. Spread the cheese sauce thinly using a spatula, about 1.5mm. It will require two trays.
4. Dry at 46° C for about 16-18 hours in the dehydrator.
5. Take the trays out to flip the sheets of cheese strokes.
6. Pick up the cheese-covered silicon sheets off of the trays. Line the trays with new silicon sheets. Flip the silicon sheets with the cheese strokes upside down and place on top of the new sheets. Carefully peel off the top silicon sheets from the cheese strokes.
7. Put back into the dehydrator for another 6 hours until completely dry.
8. Once dry, break into small shards.

Assembly

1. Place ricotta ball in the middle of the plate.
2. Carefully place sun dried tomato shards on the top of the ricotta ball in the aesthetic way (as seen on page 70).
3. Sprinkle some red cabbage microgreens and edible gold powder for a luxury look if desired. Serve!

HARD AGED TOMATO CHEESE

Time - 2-3 days

Serves - 4-6

Ingredients

140 g sunflower seeds soaked
100 g almonds peeled soaked
5 g acidophilus probiotic
1/4 cup filtered water + more as needed
4 tbsp nutritional yeast
8 pieces sundried tomatoes
2 tbsp lemon juice
2 tsp licorice salt
2 tbsp paprika for coating

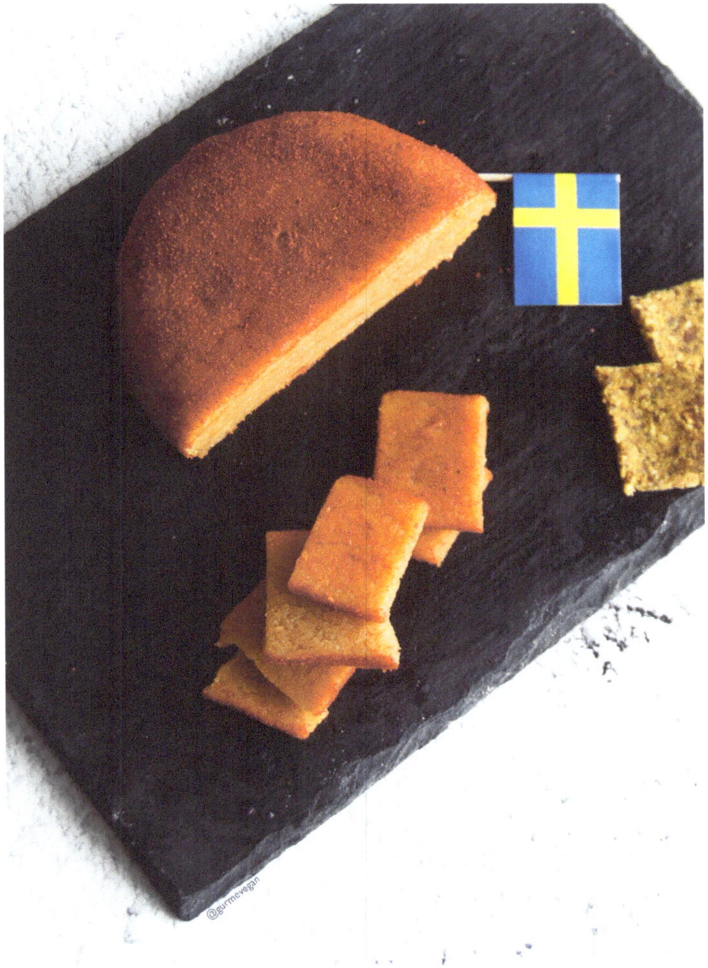

Instructions

1. Soak the sunflower seeds and almonds together in slightly warm water for 3-4 hours, then rinse and place in the food processor. Add the rest of the ingredients. Blend on high speed, scraping down the sides from time to time until you get smooth texture. In this period if you need, add more water but avoid adding too much. The consistency should not be too soft.
2. Transfer the your mixture into a cheesecloth and pull it tight. Add a weight above it and let sit at dehydrator for about 24 hours to drain possible excess water.
3. The next day, the mixture should have a slightly sour, lemony taste, like fresh cream cheese. Transfer to a spring pan, cover with plastic film to touch and place in the refrigerator for about 6 hours. After 6 hours, remove the cheese from the springform pans and place it on a plate or small baking sheet lined with parchment paper. Salt both sides with about 1/4 tsp of salt and paprika. Place in the refrigerator for 2 days.
4. As you can consume the cheese after two days, you can leave more days to age.

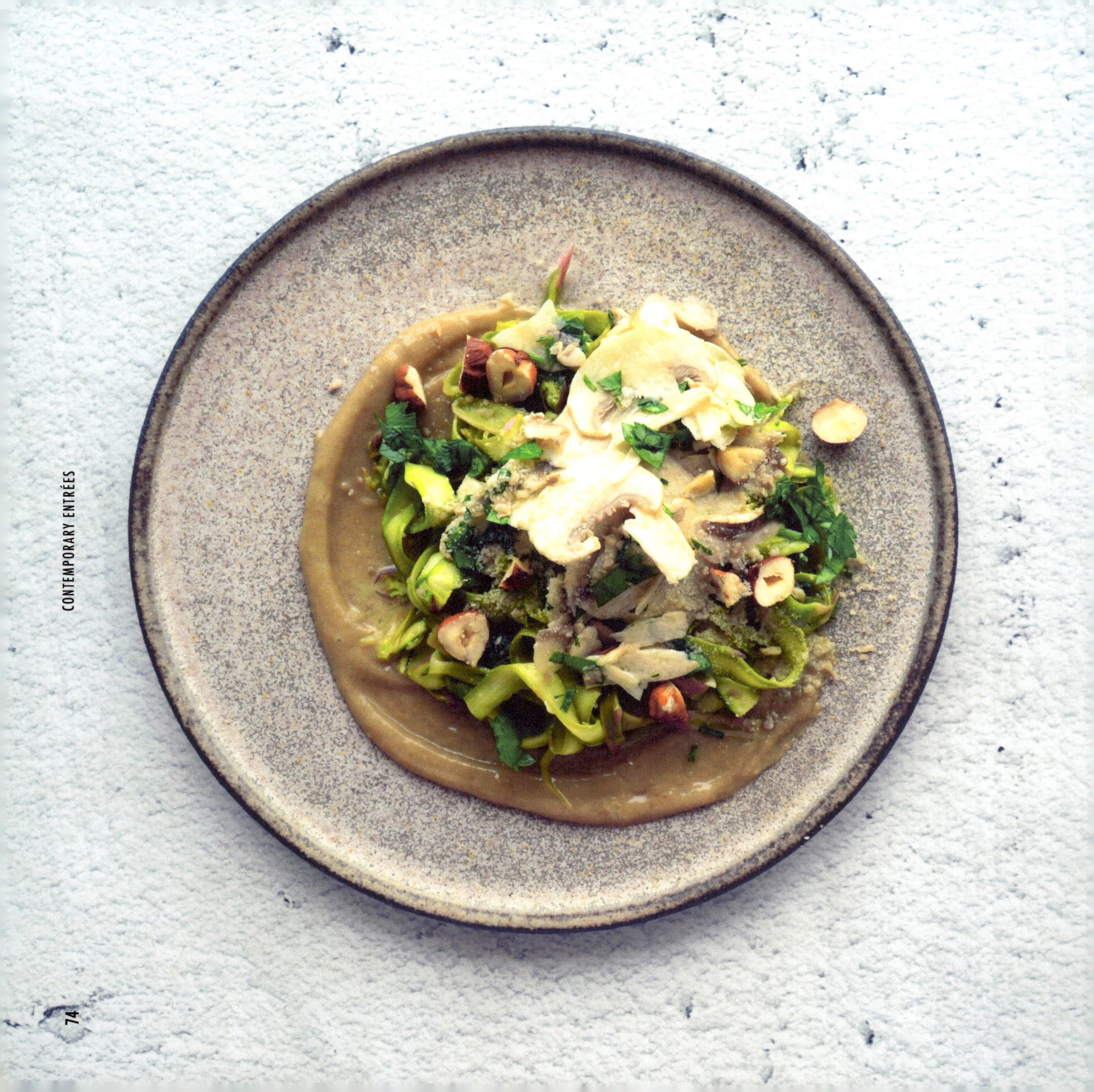

SHAVED MUSHROOM, ASPARAGUS SALAD WITH TAHINI

Category - Pure-Raw
Time - 20 minutes
Quantity- 2 plates

Equipment - Mandolin slicer
Personal note - The gorgeous medley of textures, and very complementary flavors.

Ingredients

6 stalks asparagus, ends trimmed
2 cups button mushrooms ends trimmed
2 tbsp fresh lemon juice
1 tbsp white wine vinegar
1/4 tsp salt
1 tbsp rawmesan (a mixture of nuts, nutritional yeast, salt and lemon powder)
1 tbsp crushed hazelnuts
2 tbsp tahini well-stirred
A handful parsley
Freshly ground black pepper

Instructions

1. Using a mandolin, cut the asparagus and mushrooms into paper-thin shavings.
2. In a large bowl, combine the asparagus and mushrooms and toss with the lemon juice, vinegar and salt and let stand for 5 minutes.
3. Meanwhile, stir together the tahini and about 2 tablespoons water in a small bowl until smooth.
4. Season with a pinch of salt, then using the back of a spoon, smear the mixture over your serving platter or bowl or divide it among 2 salad plates.
5. Add the olive oil and parsley to the mushrooms and gently toss to combine, then pile on top of the tahini.
6. Sprinkle with a few pinches of salt , rawmesan, crushed hazelnuts and a few grinds of black pepper. Serve immediately and eat within an hour or so, as the mushrooms start releasing liquid as the salad sits.

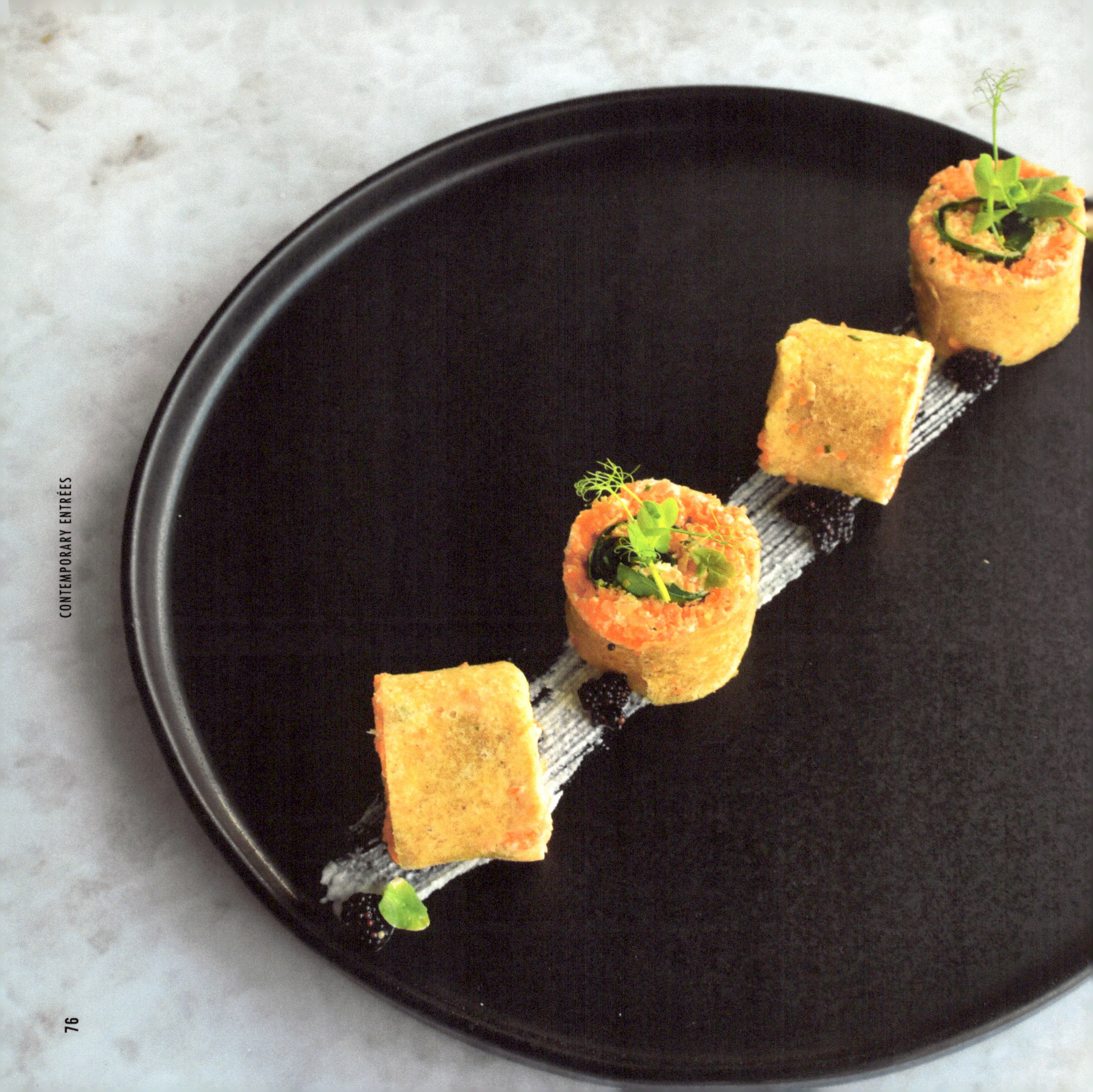

KOHLRABI CARROT ROLLS

Category - Dehydrated Raw
Preperation - 45 min + 8 hrs dehydration
Quantity - 1 wrap

Equipment - High speed blender, dehydrator, a sharp chef knife
Personal note - Like a fine dining!

Wrap Ingredients*

200 g kohlrabi peeled
1/4 cup flaxseeds
1 tbsp psyllium husk powder
1 tbsp flaxseed oil or sesame oil
1 tbsp lemon juice
1/4 tsp salt
1/2 cup water

To make kohlrabi wraps

1. Peel and wash your kohlrabi. Cut in four pieces. Add to your food processor. Pour the water. Blend until puree.
2. To have flax meal, ground flax seeds in a coffee grinder to produce a fine flour.
3. Then add the flax meal, psyllium powder, lemon juice, cold pressed sesame seed oil or flaxseed oil or olive oil and salt to your food processor. Blend until well combined.
4. Pour mixture onto a dehydrator sheet and spread evenly into a circle or square shape.
5. Dehydrate for 6-8 hours at 42° C or until able to peel off the sheet.
6. Once the nonstick sheets are removed, return to the dehydrator for 1-2 hours, until both sides are dry to the touch but still pliable. Do not dehydrate too long as breaks will occur in the wrap. You should obtain a flexible wrap and it should be easily rolled up.

* This recipe is best for a 30x30 cm dehydrator sheet and makes one large wrap. If you want to make more, double the ingredients.

kohlrabi carrot rolls continued

Almond cream cheese ingredients

60 g raw almonds soaked for 6 hrs and peeled

1 tbsp olive oil

3-4 tbsp water as needed to blend

1.5 tbsp lemon juice

1/4 tsp salt or miso

1/2 tsp minced garlic

To make almond cream cheese

1. Put soaked and peeled almonds, olive oil, garlic, salt, and water in a blender .
2. Blend until smooth and creamy, scraping down as you go. Add more water a little at a time if necessary.
3. Then add lemon juice and blend to incorporate. Taste and add salt or more lemon juice if desired.

Carrot filling ingredients

60 g carrot

1 shallot

1 tbsp lemon juice

1 tbsp fennel fronds chopped (alternatively fresh dill)

1 tbsp chopped melissa leaves

1/4 tsp salt

1 tbsp olive oil (optional)

To make carrot filling

1. In a food processor, process the carrots until broken down into a paste.
2. Add the rest of the ingredients for the carrot filling. Mix until well combined. Give it a quick squeeze with paper towel to remove a little excess moisture.

Other components

Collard greens

Black mustard caviar

Pea sprouts

Sous vide mustard caviar

1/2 cup black or yellow mustard seeds

2/3 cup white wine vinegar

1/3 cup water, plus extra for blanching

2 tbsp coconut sugar

A pinch of Salt

To make mustard caviar

1. Soak the mustard seeds in warm water for 4-5 hours and change its water every 40 minutes to release the bitter tannins from the mustard seeds.
2. Add the mustard seeds to a silicon bag and cover with enough water .
3. Using sous vide machine cook around 42° C until soft. The seeds should have almost doubled in size and have a somewhat gelatinous texture. Drain the water out by pouring the seeds into a mesh strainer and rinsing with cold water.
4. Transfer the strained seeds to a jar and add the vinegar, 1/3 cup water, coconut sugar and pinch of salt. Let it sit at room temperature for 2-3 hours then chill for at least 24 hours before serving.

Assembly

1. Lay the wrap on a work surface. Place almond cream cheese in the centre of the wrap. Spread through the middle of the wrap so that almost reaches the edges.
2. Add the carrot mixture onto the cream cheese, spread well. Add some collard greens.
3. Fold in the sides, then starting from the bottom of the wrap, roll tightly into a cylinder.
4. Cut the wrap into 4 cm thick round sections. Serve with pea sprouts and black mustard caviar if desired. Enjoy!

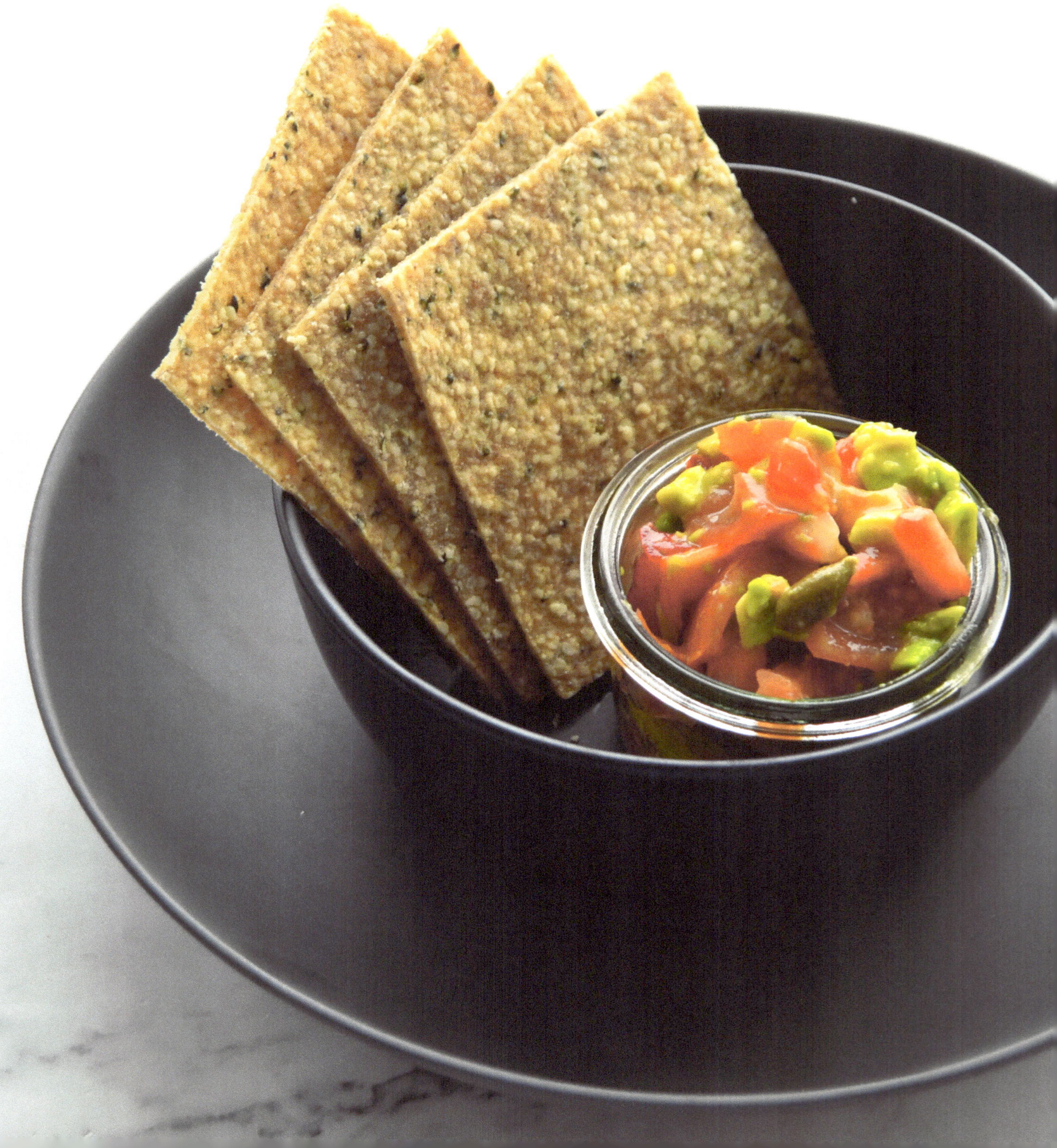

KOHLRABI HEMP SWEDISH KNÄCKEBRÖD WITH SUMMER SALSA

Category - Dehydrated- Raw

Time - 20 min prep + 24 hrs dehydration

Equipment - Blender, non-stick sheets, spatula, dehydrator, a sharp chef knife

Quantity - 1 dehydrator tray 30x30 cm

Ingredients

135 g kohlrabi

1/2 tbsp hemp oil

1 cup hemp hearts

1/4 tsp salt

1 tbsp psyllium husk

1/2 cup water

Summer salsa

1 ripe avocado

4-5 strawberries

4-5 cherry tomatoes

1 garlic cloves minced

1 tbsp capers

A pinch of salt

Instructions

1. Peel your kohlrabi, remove the skin. Cut the kohlrabi meat into chunks. Measure it and transfer 135 g of it to a high speed blender. Add the hemp oil, alternatively you can use flax-seed oil, sesame oil or olive oil. Add the water. Blend until smooth.
2. Then add the hemp hearts, salt and psyllium husk powder. Blend until combined.
3. Let it sit for 5-6 minutes until psyllium absorbs the water and it becomes a thick spreadable mixture.
4. Once done, using an offset spatula, spread the mixture thinly over the dehydrator tray lined silicon paper.
5. Dehydrate at 42° C for 10 hours, them flip the other side of the bread and continue to dehydrate. Check every 3-4 hours as much as possible and flip it.
6. To make summer salsa, peel and remove the seed of your avocado. Using a sharp knife chop finely. Transfer to a bowl. Chop tomatoes and strawberries. Add lemon juice , salt , capers and minced garlic. Combine well. Serve with your knäckebröd.

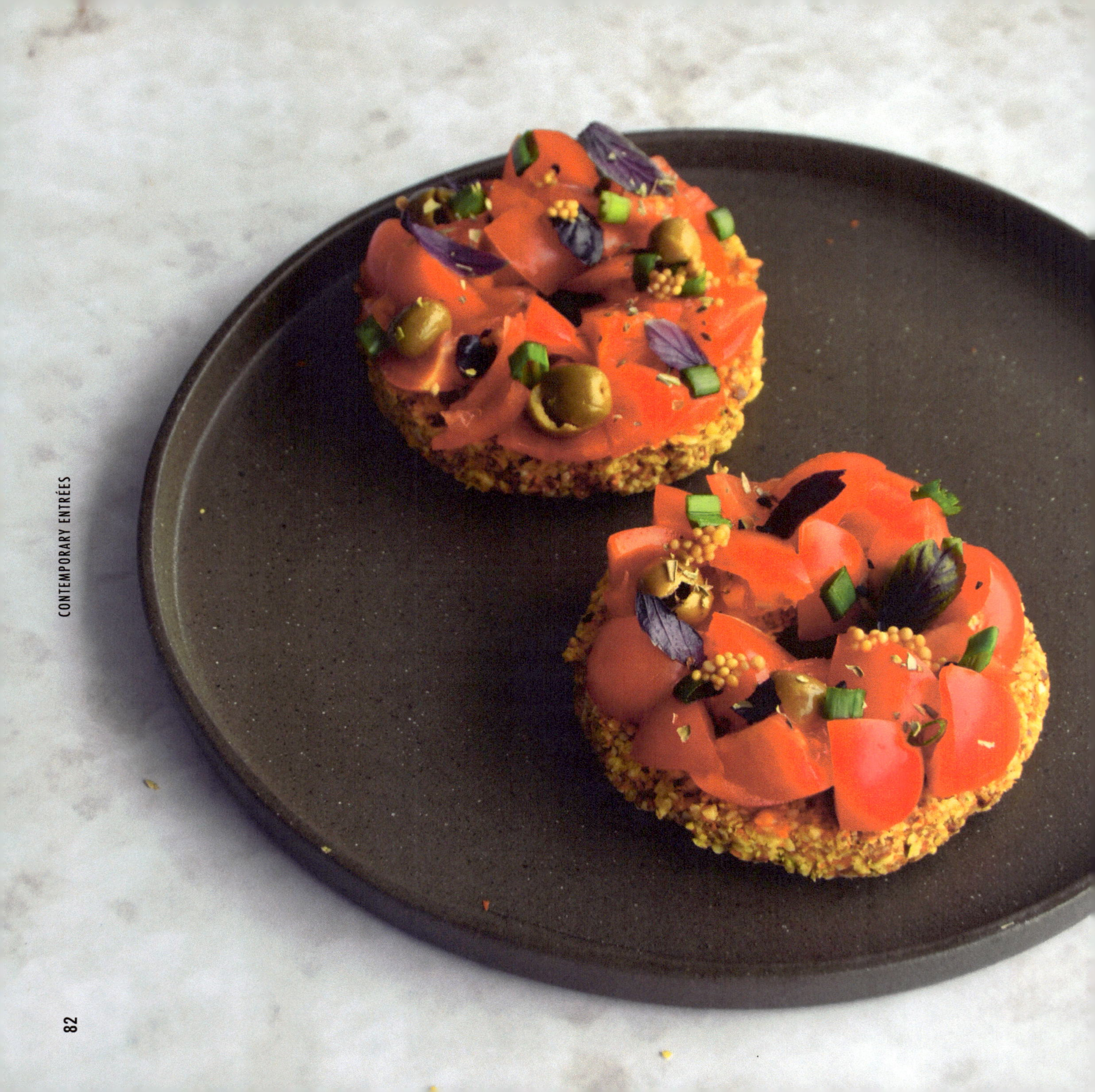

DOUBLE TOMATO BRUSCHETTA BAGELS

Category - Dehydrated-Raw
Dehydration time - 12-16 hours
Quantity - 3-4 person

Equipment - Food processor, dehydrator
Personal note - Crispy italian, perfect as a breakfast or starter.

Ingredients
1 cup almonds soaked
1 cup carrots shredded
4 springs green onions
3 tbsp ground flaxseeds
2 tbsp apple cider vinegar
2 tbsp extra virgin olive oil
1/2 tsp sea salt
2 tbsp water

Toppings:
Fresh tomatoes chopped
Green olives
Green onion chopped
Fresh basil
Pickled mustard seeds

Instructions
1. Place the soaked almonds and carrots together with the vinegar, olive oil, flax, garlic, spring onions and sea salt to your food processor. Process until a sticky dough forms. You will need to keep scraping down the sides of your processor.
2. Add 2-3 tbsp water. If dough isn't quite workable, shape it with your hands carefully.
3. Form into rolls, a bit thicker than the size of bagel you want, and mush the edges together to form the shape of a bagel.
4. Sprinkle the top, and sides with sesame seeds, lightly pressing them in.
5. Dehydrate at 46° C until the top is slightly dry, flip over and sprinkle with more seeds, pressing them in.
6. Dehydrate another hour or so and flip back over. Then leave overnight or roughly 8-9 hours. Serve with tomatoes, pickled mustards seeds, chives and green olives or whatever you like.

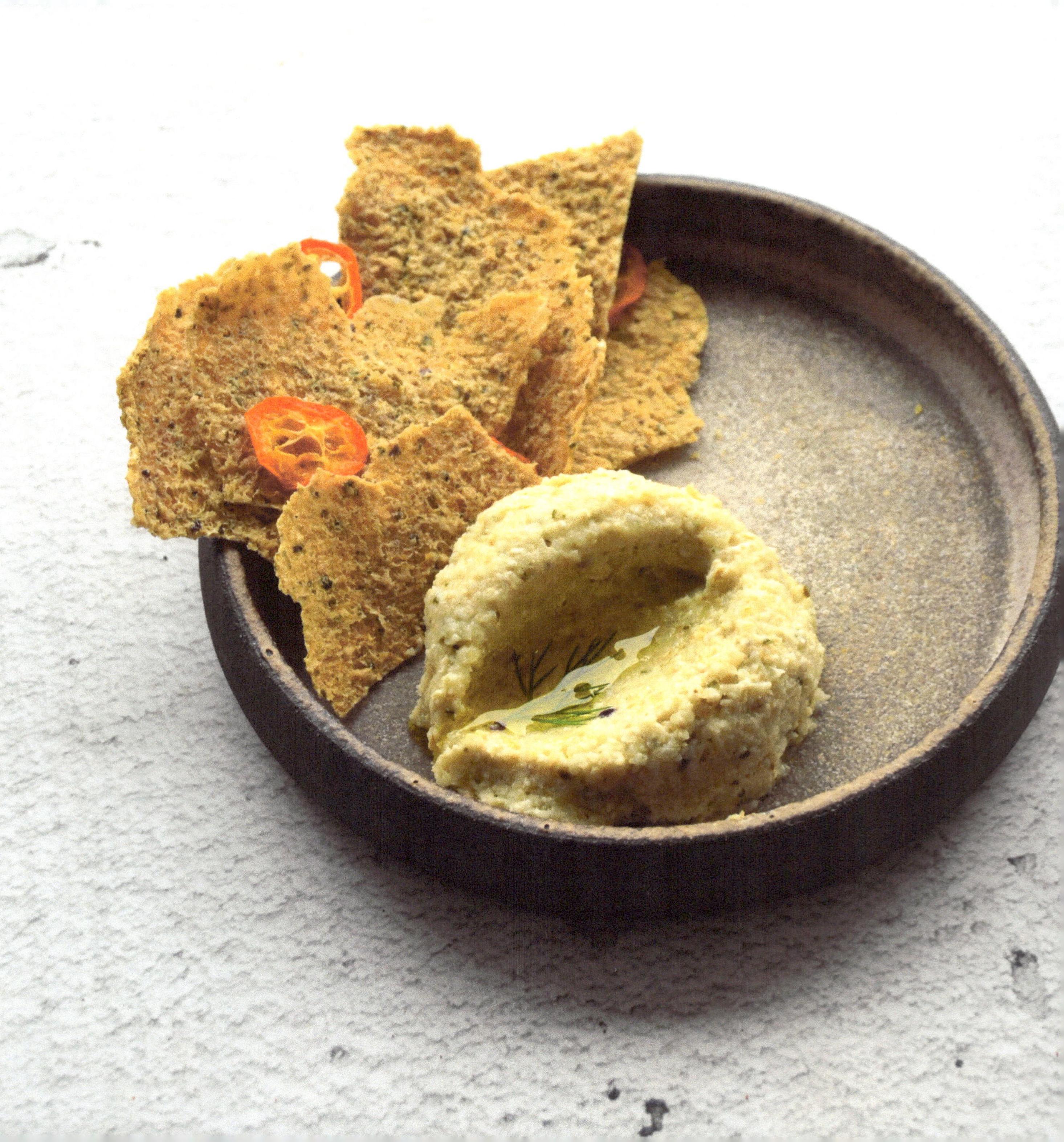

SAVE THE FISH PATE AND BRITTLE

Category - Sous-Vide + Dehydrated-Raw
Preperation - 30 min + 3 hrs sous vide + 6 hrs dehydration
Quantity - 2 person

Ingredients

250 g fresh artichoke hearts (alternatively heart of palm, jackfruit or celery root)
1/3 cup sprouted oat flour
1/4 cup water
2 tbsp lemon juice
1 tsp coconut aminos (or 1/2 tsp tamari)
1/2 tsp seaweed blend (from Lofoten Seaweed)
Salt and black pepper to taste
2 tsp onion powder

Equipment - Food processor, dehydrator, sous-vide, spatula
Personal note - Versatile plant based sea food flavours, both brittle and pâté made of same mixture.

Seaweed blend

Dulse
Atlantic Wakame
Winged Kelp

Instructions

1. Cook the artichoke hearts sous vide. Sous vide artichoke root usually needs 2-3 hours at 46° C to become tender. Peel it, then cut into rounds or cube before placing in a single layer in the sous vide bag. Once soften, transfer to the food processor.
2. In a food processor combine all the ingredients. Pulse a few times until ingredients are broken down, well combined and smooth. If you will make pâté, just serve with the bread or crackers. Keep in the refrigerator up to 2-3 days. It is best when consumed in the same day.
3. To make brittle, spread mixture thinly over the dehydrator tray lined silicon paper. Sprinkle some extra seaweed if you like.
4. Then dehydrate at 42° C for 5-6 hours or until completely dried.

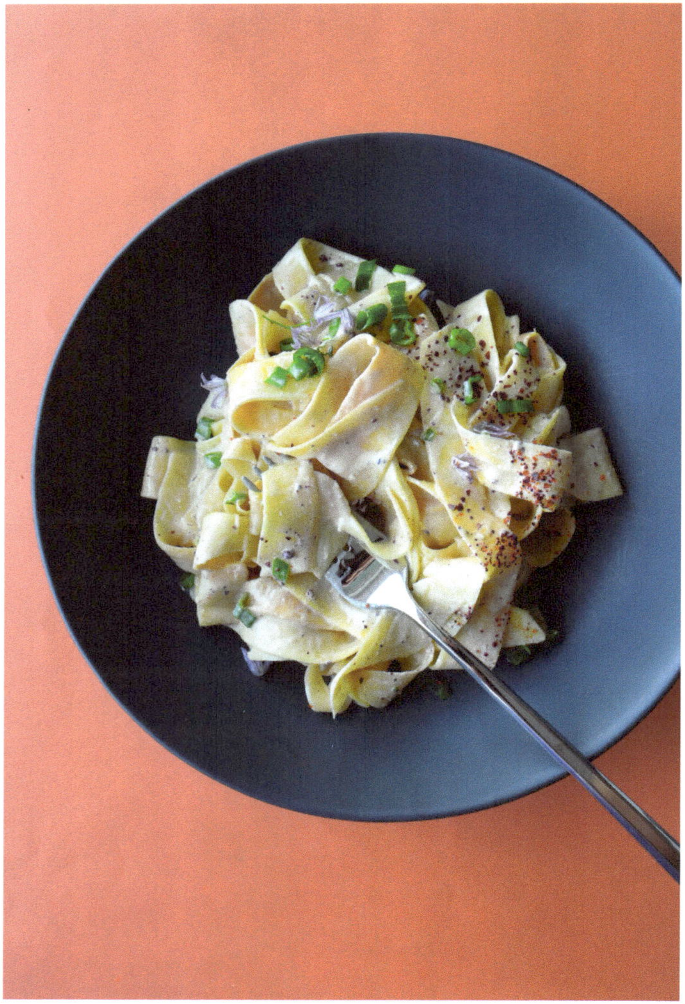

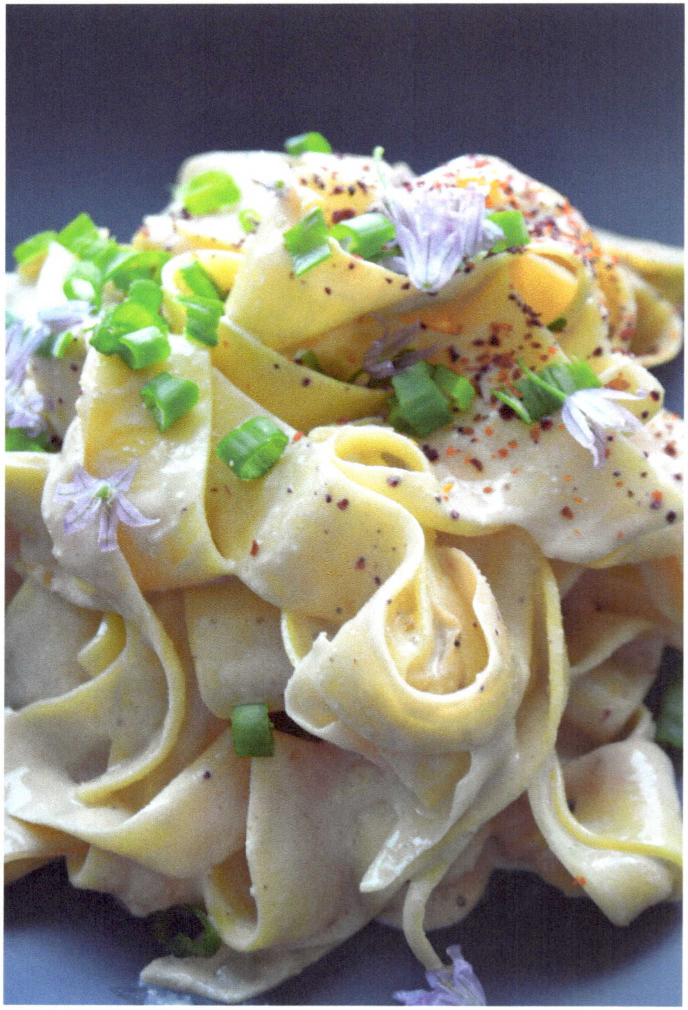

GREEN PAPAYA TAGLIATELLE

Category - Pure-Raw
Time -20 minutes
Quantity - 2 person

Ingredients
1 large green papaya
100 g almonds soaked and peeled
1 tbsp olive oil
100 ml water + more if you need to blend
3 tbsp lemon juice
2 cloves garlic minced
1 tsp miso or salt
1 tsp sumac
1 tsp chili
Chive blossoms to serve
Chopped spring onions to serve

Equipment - Mandoline slicer
Note - You probably wonder what is the difference between green papaya and papaya. Though very different in taste, texture, and appearance, green and orange papaya are actually the same fruit picked at different stages of development.

Green papaya ripens when kept next to an apple for 3 days at room temperature, it is not as sweet as regular papaya, its taste is slightly cucumber-like and slightly sweet.

Instructions
1.To make papaya tagliatelle, cut off the tough ends of the green papaya and peel the skin. Split them and remove the seeds from it if has (some green papayas have no seeds inside). Use a vegetable peeler or mandolin to trim the green papaya into tagliatelle shape.
2. Place soaked and peeled almonds in high speed blender, add the lemon juice, olive oil, garlic, miso or salt, sumac, chili and some water to blender. Mix on high speed until you get smooth mixture. Taste it, adjust the seasoning, add more salt and pepper if you wish.
3.Pour the sauce over the papaya pasta. Massage with your hands well. Cover the bowl and keep in the refrigerator for 1 hour until softened and ready to be eaten. Serve with nut parmesan if desired.
4.Once done, serve with chive blossoms and spring onions.

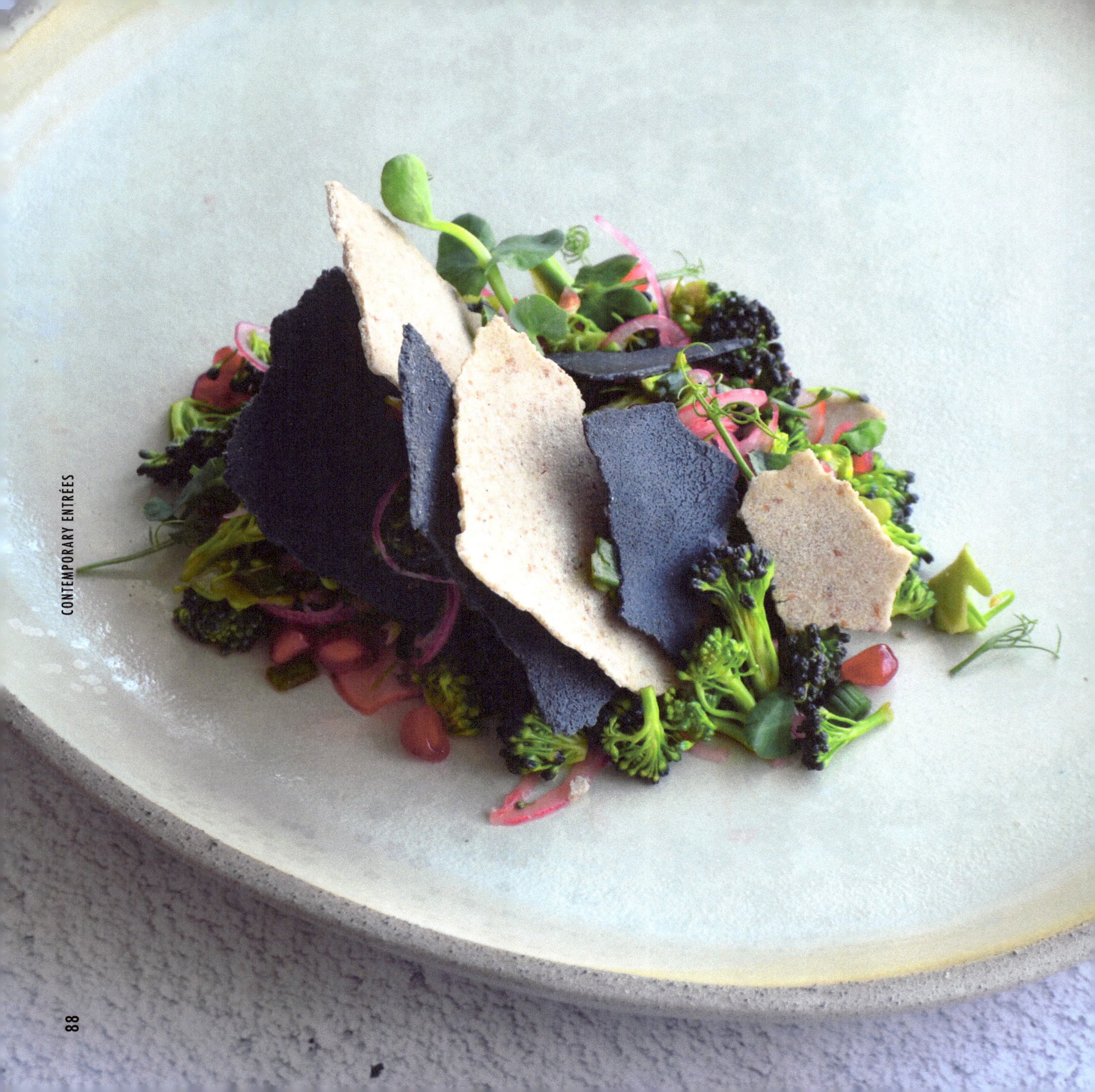

BROCCOLI SALAD WITH ROSEMARY BUCKWHEAT BRITTLE

Category - Dehydrated-Raw + Pure-Raw
Time - 20 min prep + 8 hrs dehydration

Equipment -Food processor, dehydrator
Quantity - 2 person

Ingredients

1 cup chopped broccoli
1/4 cup pomegranate
A few pea sprouts
2 small thinly sliced radish
2-3 springs green onions chopped
2 tbsp red onions thinly sliced
1 ripe avocado
3 tbsp lemon juice

Buckwheat brittle

1 cup raw buckwheat groats
1/2 cup almonds
1 cup coconut milk
1 tsp garlic powder
1 tsp dried rosemary
1/2 tsp salt
1 tsp charcoal powder (optional if you want black colored)

Instructions for the brittle

1.To make brittle, Pour buckwheat groats and almonds into separate bowls and cover with water. Soak for at least 1 hour or preferably overnight.
2. Transfer soaked buckwheat groats to a colander. Thoroughly rinse and drain. Repeat the process for the almonds too.
3. Combine all the ingredients in a blender and then process at high speed until smooth.
4. Spread the buckwheat on dehydrator trays covered with non-stick silicon sheets or parchment paper. Dry at 42°C for 8-10 hours until you get brittle.

Instructions for the broccoli salad

1. Wash and drain your broccoli florets. Finely chop using a sharp knife. Add to a bowl.
2. Using a mandoline slicer, thinly slice radish and red onions. Add onto the broccoli.
3. Add the sliced green onion, pea sprouts, lemon juice and pomegranate seeds. Toss well.
4. In a small food processor, blend avocado with salt and lemon juice until smooth.
5. Pour sauce on to the plate. Add your salad on the sauce.
6. Randomly break the buckwheat brittle, serve with your salad.

CRISPY BROCCOLI BALLS

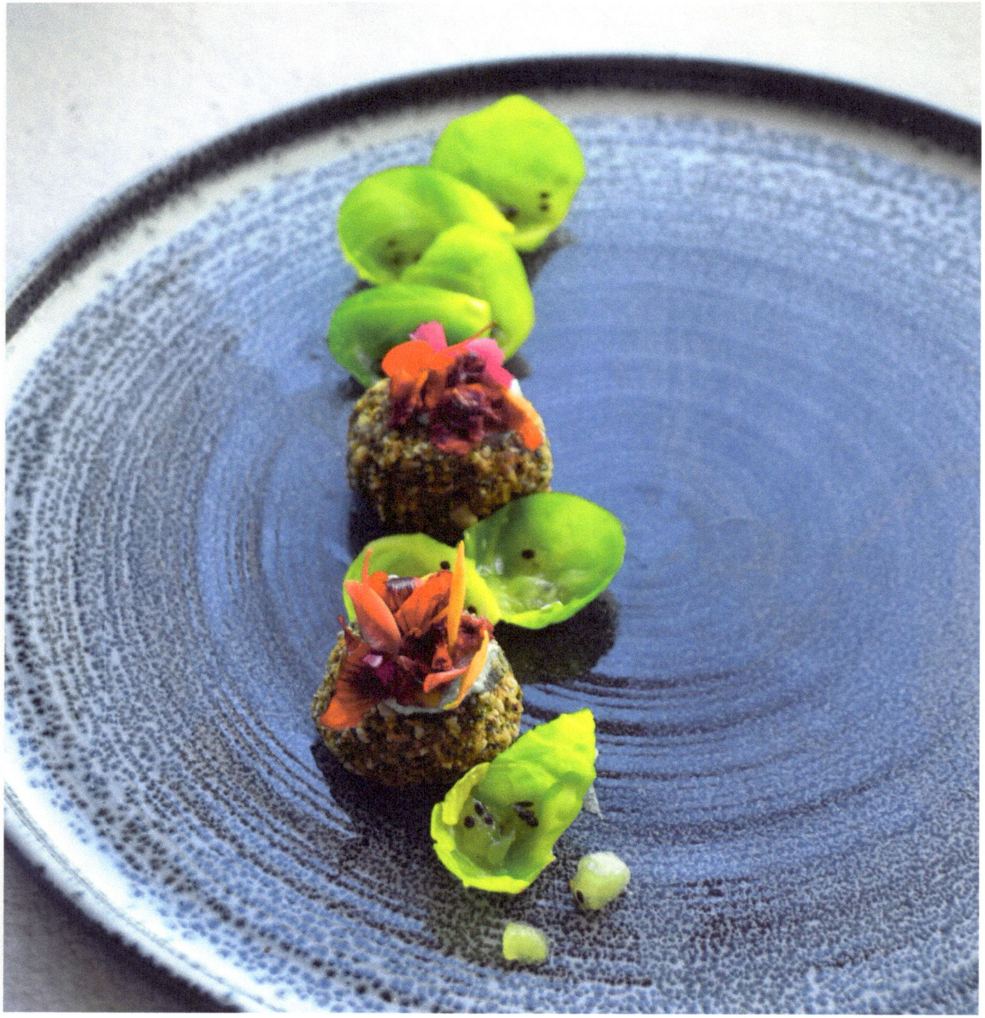

These are a great protein hit, a great blood purifier, and loads of fiber as well. Our addition to these great balls is, serving with seed cheese cream, massaged brussels sprouts and kiwi sauce.

Category - Dehydrated-Raw
Time - 15 min + 14 hrs dehydration
Serves - 8-12 balls

Equipment - Food processor, dehydrator
Personal note - Experimental

Ingredients
260 g broccoli chopped
1/2 cup sunflower seeds soaked
1/2 cup flaxmeal
1/4 cup onion chopped
2 garlic cloves minced
2 tbsp parsley chopped
2 tbsp nutritional yeast
1 tbsp olive oil
1/2 tsp salt

Instructions
1. Place all ingredients in a processor and blend until well mixed.
2. Transfer mixture into a bowl.
3. Scoop out a spoonful, roll into a ball with hands.
4. Repeat until you have used all the mix.
5. Dehydrate for 12-14 hours or overnight before serving.

This can be served with a small salad, preferred sauce, or add into a pasta dish.

Optional
If you want to experiment with kiwi sauce and brussels sprouts, simply mix 1/2 cup kiwi with 1 tbsp lemon juice and 1/2 tbsp maple. Massage brussels sprouts with salt and apple cider vinegar. Serve together.

SAMOSA

Category - Dehydrated-Raw
Dehydration time - 5 hours
Serves - 2 person

Equipment - Food processor, blender, dehydrator, a sharp chef knife
Storage - In the refrigerator up to 2 months.

Samosa dough ingredients

2 medium rutabaga peeled
2 medium red apple peeled
3 tbsp chopped onion
3 tbsp olive oil
3 tbsp psyllium husk powder
1 cup water
1/4 tsp sea salt

Instructions

1. To prepare the samosa mixture, in a high–speed blender or food processor, blend all ingredients, except the psyllium husk powder, until smooth. Place mixture into a bowl.
2. Add the psyllium husk powder and combine to the consistency of thin paste.
3. On silicon dehydrator sheets, spread mixture in a thin layer, just under 3mm thick, and place in the dehydrator at 46°C for 4-5 hrs.
4. Once the mixture is well set, but not completely dry, loosen the edges with a knife and invert directly onto a screen. Finish dehydrating until the backs are dry. Check often. You do not want to over dry the crêpes or they will not stay pliable.

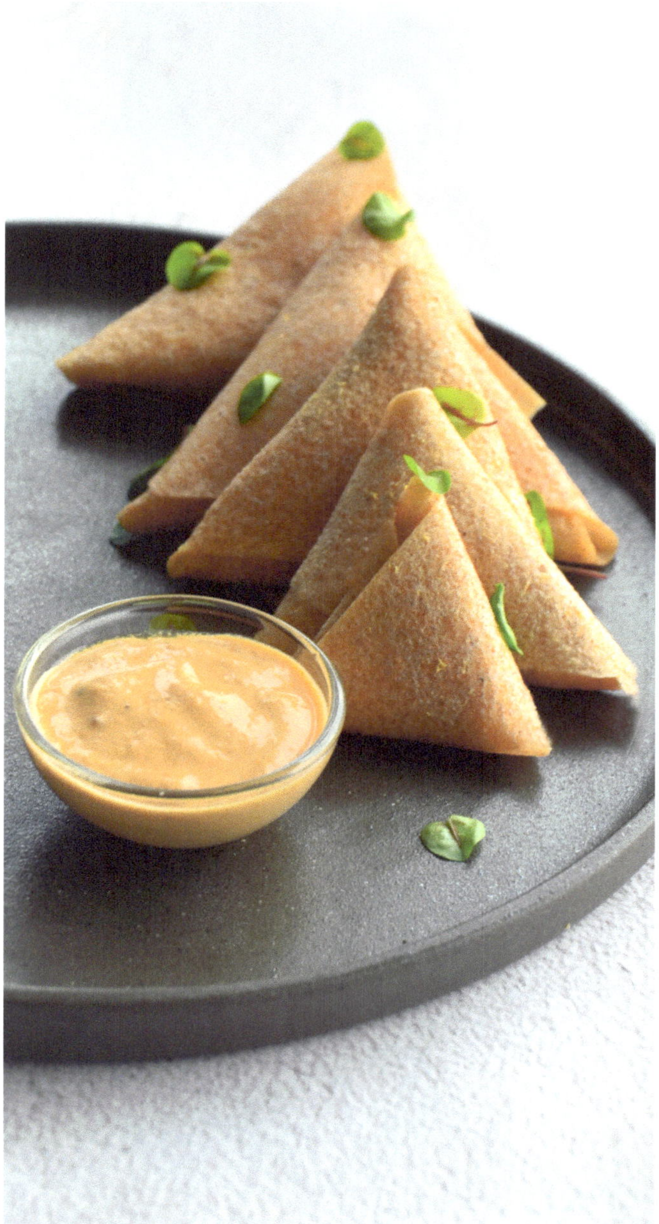

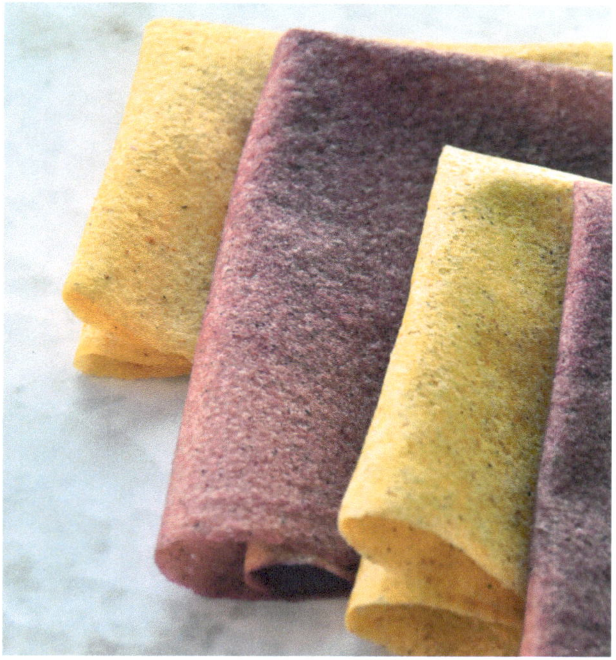

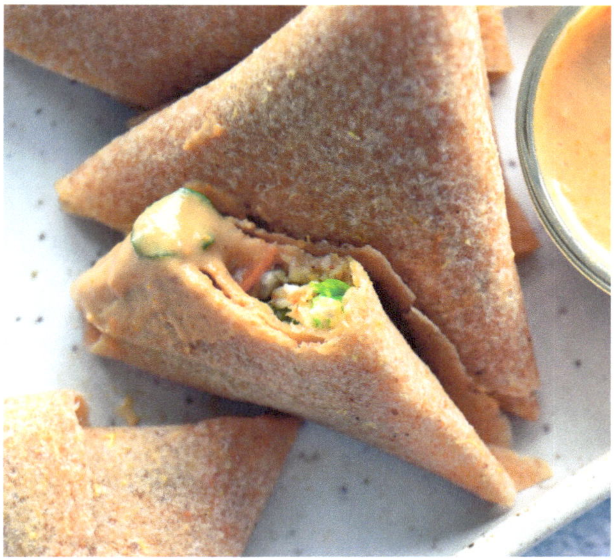

Samosa continued

Filling ingredients

60 g cauliflower riced

40 g sunflower seeds

50 g sweet peas

2 small red bell pepper diced

30 g carrots diced

2 tbsp olive oil

1/2 tbsp fresh ginger grated

1 shallot chopped

1 tsp garlic clove minced

2 tbsp lemon juice

1/2 tsp salt

To make filling

1. In a food processor, pulse the cauliflower with the sunflower seeds until a finely-minced consistency. Transfer to a mixing bowl.
2. Add the remaining ingredients and thoroughly combine.

Curry sauce Ingredients

40 g sun-dried tomatoes

2 tbsp tahini

1/2 tsp ginger powder

A pinch clove powder

1 tsp curry powder

1 tsp mustard powder

3 tbsp lemon juice

120 ml water

1/2 tsp salt

to make curry sauce

1. Add all the ingredients to your blender. Blend well until you get smooth mixture.
2. Place in the fridge for 2 hours before serving, it will get thicker.

Assembly

1. Slice each samosa dough into 7-8cm strips. Lay out the strips on surface, add about 2 tbsp of samosa filling on the end of each and continue to fold into samosa–size triangles.
2. Place the filled triangles on a dehydrator sheet and dry at 46°C for 45-50 minutes before serving.
3. Serve with curry sauce .

Notes

As raw food recipes will always turn out different for everyone depending on the ingredient, dehydrator you have and experience, it's best to start paying attention to consistency, which is really one of the most important aspects of working with raw food recipes. You don't want the mixture to be too runny or too firm, just a nice spreadable batter. If you think it's looking too thick, start by adding 2 tbsp water and work your way up from there.

Tips

To make yellow samosas, add 1/2 tsp turmeric to dough mixture, for the pink color add beet powder or replace water with fresh beet juice.

nostalgic mains

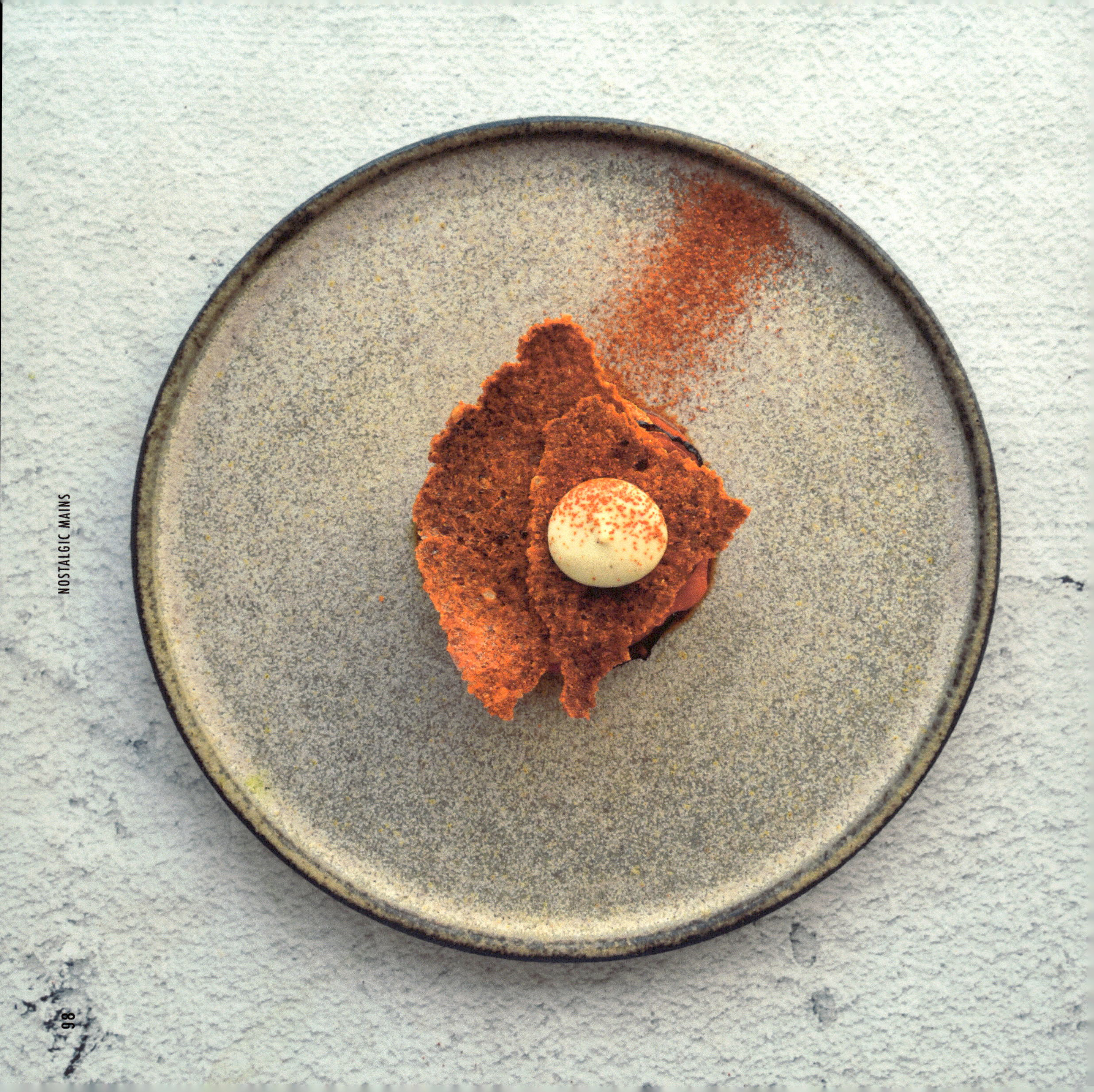

RAWATOUILLE

Category - Dehydrated-Raw
Time - 45 min prep + 5 hrs dehydration

Equipment - Food processor, mandoline slicer, dehydrator, piping bag
Quantity - 4-6 person

Ingredients

2 red onions
2 aubergines
3 courgettes
2 red peppers
6 tomatoes
15 g fresh thyme
A few springs of green onions
2 tbsp lemon juice

Tomato Sauce

400 g shredded tomatoes
2 tbsp olive oil
2 tbsp balsamic vinegar
10g chopped basil
4 cloves of garlic
Black pepper and salt to taste

Instructions

1. Peel the onions, aubergines and courgettes. Using a mandoline slicer, slice them thinly. Deseed the peppers and chop thinly. Using a sharp knife slice the tomatoes too.
2. While you are making the sauce, place all the sliced veggies in a bowl, add lemon juice and cold water with ice cubes in order to prevent them from getting brown.
3. To make the tomato sauce, pick the basil leaves and set aside, then finely slice the stalks. Peel and mince the garlic. Stir them in the fresh shredded tomatoes, olive oil, the balsamic and a good pinch of sea salt and black pepper. Mix well.
4. Remove vegetable slices from the water. Place in a large bowl. Pour the tomato sauce over the veggies. Massage well. Cover bowl and let it marinate for 1-2 hours.

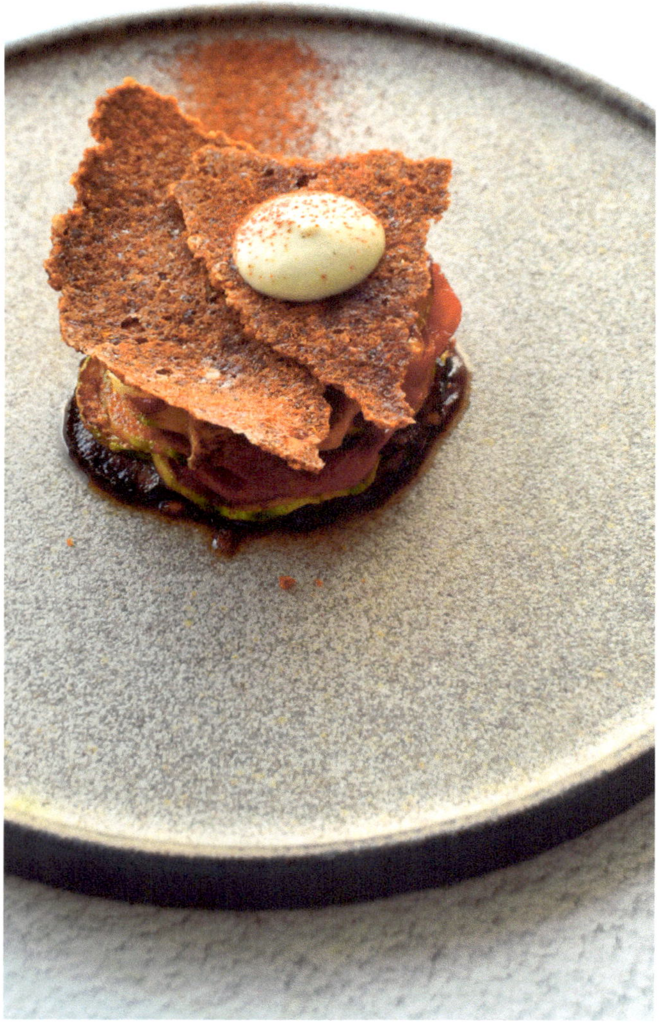

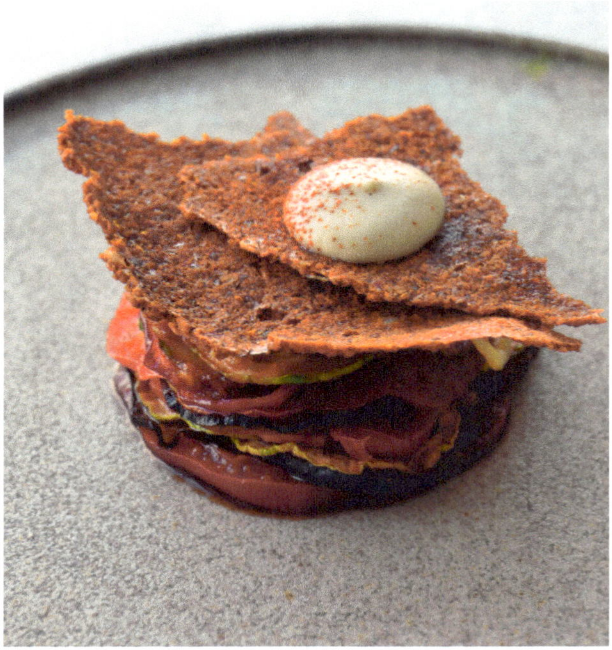

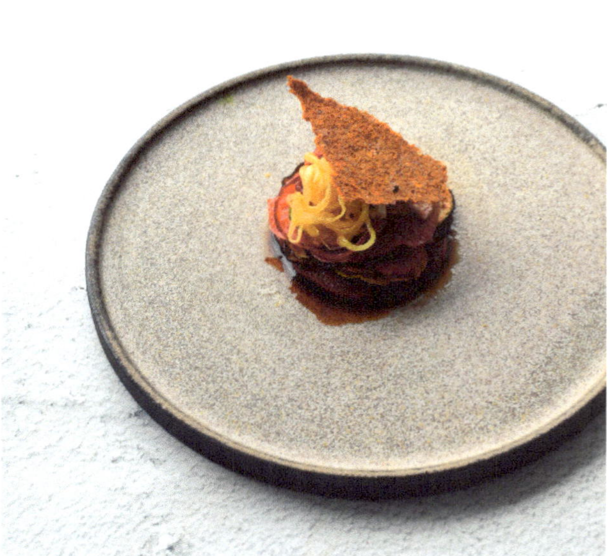

5. Once marinated, carefully place the sliced vegetables onto the dehydrator trays lined silicon baking sheet. Keep a distance between them so that they overlap.
6. Dehydrate at 42° C for 3-4 hours. Monitor them during the process, we want them semi-soft, not crispy like chips.
7. Once soften, remove from the dehydrator. If you want a spiral stack for presentation like ratatouille, layer sliced semi-soft vegetables in a pyrex and serve in this way.

Notes: Slicing all the veggies super thin is key to make a good looking ratatouille. Use mandoline slicer. This also ensures everything cooks evenly.

So far, we talked about the classic ratatouille making. Accompanied by dehydrated tomato crackers, bechamel sauce and miso glazed, ratatouille will make your guests feel more than just an ordinary meal.

If you take your guests to the atmosphere in this photo, continue with the steps below.

Miso Glaze
1 tbsp light miso
1 tbsp coconut aminos or tamari
1/2 tbsp rice vinegar
1/2 tbsp maple
1/8 tsp chili flakes
1/8 tsp salt

Instructions for the miso glaze

That's full of irresistible flavor, umami-packed glaze is perfect for vegetables, not only ratatouille, you can use for any kind of vegetable dish.
All you have to do is whisk the ingredients together and voila: instant miso glaze! One note is that you may find that there are a few chunks of miso that do not dissolve: that's ok! Just try to get it as smooth as you can.

Béchamel Sauce

1 cup cashews
1 + 1/4 cup water
2 tbsp gf nutritional yeast
2 cloves garlic
1 tbsp onion granules
1/4 tsp freshly grated nutmeg
A pinch white pepper
1 tbsp olive oil
1/2 tsp pinch salt

Instructions for the béchamel

1. In a medium bowl, soak the cashews in water for 3 to 4 hours to soften.
2. Transfer to a high speed blender. Add the rest of the ingredients.
3. Blend well until silky smooth. Add more liquid if you choose to have a thinner consistency and continue to blend. We can recommend to use a Blendtec with the twister jar. It makes everything easier.

Storage: Cashew béchamel will keep for a few day in the refrigerator and can be frozen for up to 3 months or so. After freezing it may be a bit lumpy or just not as smooth, so you might need to re-blend to smooth it out and bring it back together.

Tomato crackers

200 g tomatoes

1/2 cup flaxseeds

1/2 tbsp coconut aminos

1/4 tsp salt

1/4 tsp dried thyme

Instructions for the tomato crackers

1. Put all ingredients in a food processor and process.
2. Scoop dough onto dehydrator tray lined silicon sheets, and spread it out with a spatula in large squares about 1/2 cm thick.
3. Score dough with a spatula or knife into crackers shapes.
4. Dehydrate at 42 °C for 4-6 hours. Flip crackers and dehydrate for another 4 hours or until desired crunchiness is attained.

Other components

1 tsp paprika or tomato powder for plating.

Assembly

1. Using a tablespoon, pour 2 tbsp miso glaze in the middle of your plate.
2. Place ratatouille on the miso glaze.
3. Break a large piece from tomato crackers, top on the ratatouille.
4. Transfer béchamel sauce into a piping bag, pipe onto the tomato cracker.
5. Using a tea strainer, dust some paprika or tomato powder over the béchamel.
6. Serve immediately.

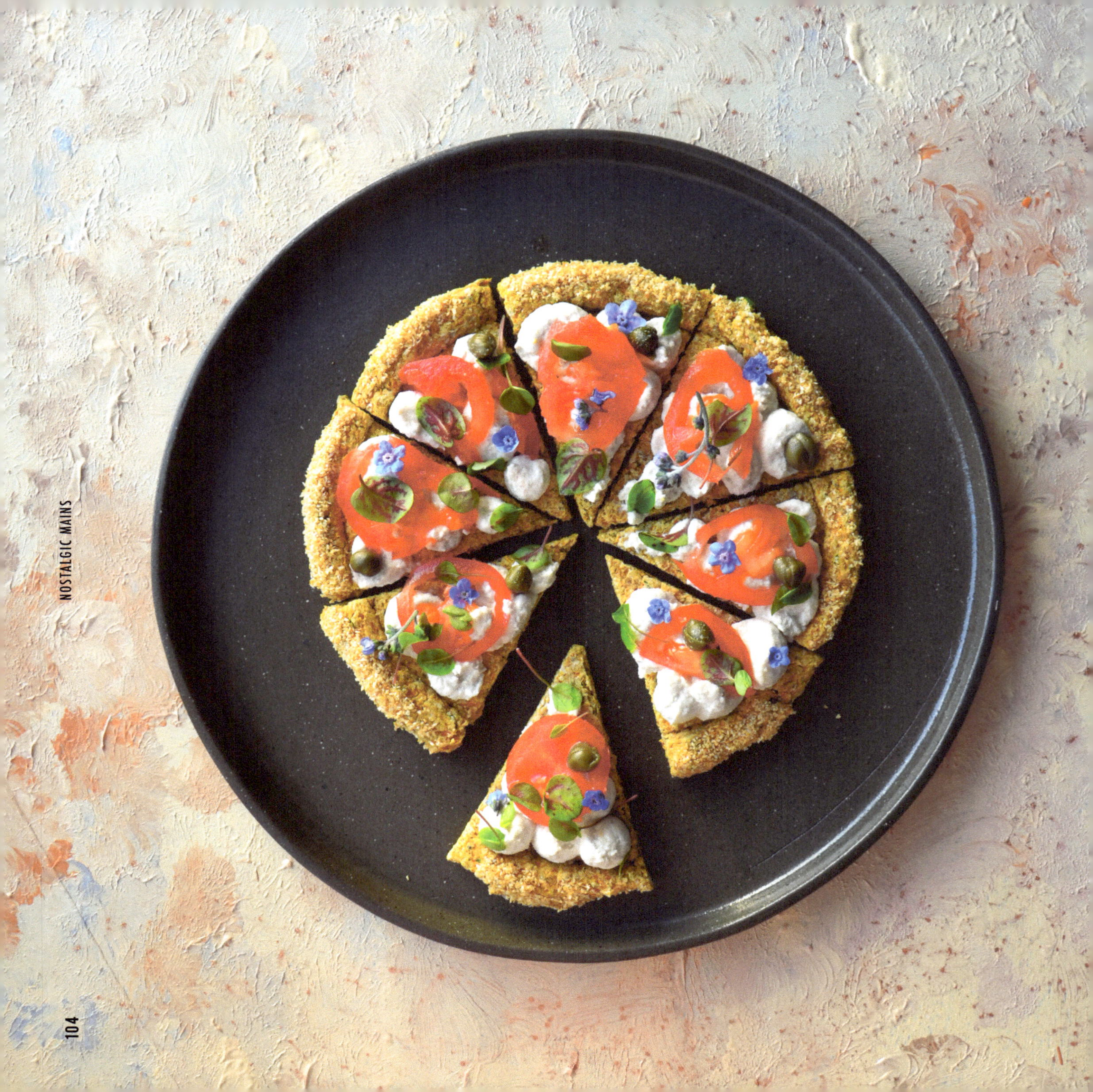

FORGET ME NOT PIZZA

Category - Dehydrated-Raw
Time - 20 min prep + 16 hrs dehydration
Quantity - 2 X 15 cm pizza

Equipment - Food processor, dehydrator, piping bag, 15 cm round cake mould to cut
Personal note - Spring feelings

Crust ingredients

1 cup sprouted dehydrated buckwheat
250 g pumpkin chopped
2 tbsp spring onions chopped
2 tbsp chia seeds
1 tbsp psyllium husk powder
1 tbsp olive oil
1 tbsp coconut sugar
1/2 tsp salt
1 tbsp garlic granules for the edges

Instructions

1. Add sprouted and dehydrated buckwheats in the food processor, blend until you get fine powder.
2. Chop pumpkin in a food processor. Add to your blender. Then add the rest of the ingredients except garlic granules. Blend well.
3. Let it set in the food processor for 10-15 minutes for the psyllium and chia to absorb the water content from the pumpkin. If your pumpkin has no juice, you may need to add 2-3 tbsp water.
4. When it is done, Divide the dough in two and make a ball. Place a dough ball between two baking paper, roll it out in a circle of about 18-20 cm using a rolling pin. Then use a 15cm round cake mold to make a ring out of the dough. Transfer the dough to your dehydrator tray lined silicon sheet.
5.Edge your pizza by shaping the remaining edges lengthwise with your hand. Turn the edges round the pizza. Sprinkle garlic powder over the edges.
6. Repeat the process for the remaining dough. You can make grissini from the leftover dough, cover with sesame and bake.
7. Dehydrate for 12-16 hours at 42°C.

forget me not pizza continued

Seed cheese cream ingredients

1 cup sunflower seeds

4 tbsp lemon juice

1/2 cup water

1 tsp salt

2 tbsp gluten free nutritional yeast (optional)

To make seed cheese cream

1. Blend everything in the food processor until smooth.
2. Keep in the refrigerator for 2-3 hours before using.

Toppings

1/4 cup cherry tomatoes

1 tbsp capers

Forget me not flowers to decorate

Vene cress, basil or oregano

Extra virgin olive oil to drizzle if desired

Assembly

1. Spread a thin layer of seed cheese cream on the crust , alternatively, pour the cheese in a piping bag and drop cheese dots over the crust.
2. Add the capers, cherry tomatoes and herbs. Decorate with forget me not flowers.
3. Drizzle some olive oil if desired.
4. You can eat it fresh or dehydrator for 1-2 hours before eating.

PASTA AL POMODORO

Category - Dehydrated-Raw
Dehydration time - 5 hours
Serves - 4 person

Pasta dough ingredients
400 g fresh heirloom corn
1/2 cup water
2 tbsp psyllium husk powder
1 tsp salt

Equipment - Food processor, dehydrator
Personal note - A real chewy pasta feeling! This satisfying new experience will make pasta lovers feel nostalgia.
Storage - in the refrigerator up to 2 months.

Instructions
1. Place the fresh corns to your blender. Add the water and salt. Blend until smooth.
2. Then add the psyllium husk, blend again till combined well.
3. Let it sit for 10 minutes until psyllium absorbs the water.
4. When the dough has come together smoothly, if it's feeling moist, incorporate some more psyllium husk into the dough. You want to end up with a ball that's not too sticky, but still soft.
5. Roll the dough between parchment paper and roll them out until it is about 1.5mm thick. (200 g dough per 30x30 cm dehydrator tray)
6. Place dough to your dehydrator sheet lined parchment paper. Dehydrate for 1-2 hours at 42° C until it becomes easily reversible.
7. At this stage you will shape your pasta dough. Cut into desired shape. To make farfalle, take your ravioli wheel cutter and cut the rectangle into strips. Your strips should be approximately 4-5cm wide and 2cm long.

8. Use your thumb and forefinger to pinch the long edges together to form a bow.
9. Repeat with remaining rectangles, then remaining pieces of dough. Arrange the pasta in a single layer on dehydrator sheet. Ensure there is a good amount of space between each shape to avoid them from sticking together.
10. Dehydrate for 1 hour then combine with your sauce and eat. If you want to consume later, dehydrate for 4-5 hours or until completely dried and store in the airtight container.

Rawmesan ingredients

1 cup pine nuts
2 tbsp nutritional yeast
1/4 tsp lemon powder
1/2 tsp salt

To make rawmesan

1. Place all ingredients into your blender.
2. Blend well until combined.

Tomato sauce ingredients

1 cup fresh heirloom tomatoes
1/2 cup sundried tomatoes
2 tsp coconut sugar
1 tbsp garlic minced
3 tbsp extra virgin olive oil
Salt to taste

To make tomato sauce

1. Place all ingredients to your blender.
2. Blend well until puree.
3. Transfer in a bowl. Dehydrate for 2-3 hours at 46° C until become thick and warm. If the tomatoes are too juicy, you may want to strain the water or add some chia seeds to obtain a thick consistency.

Assembly

1. In warm water, soak your pasta for 5-6 minutes or more as you need, then strain.
2. Toss your farfalle with the sauce. Drizzle extra virgin olive oil if desired.
3. Serve with rawmesan and edible flowers.

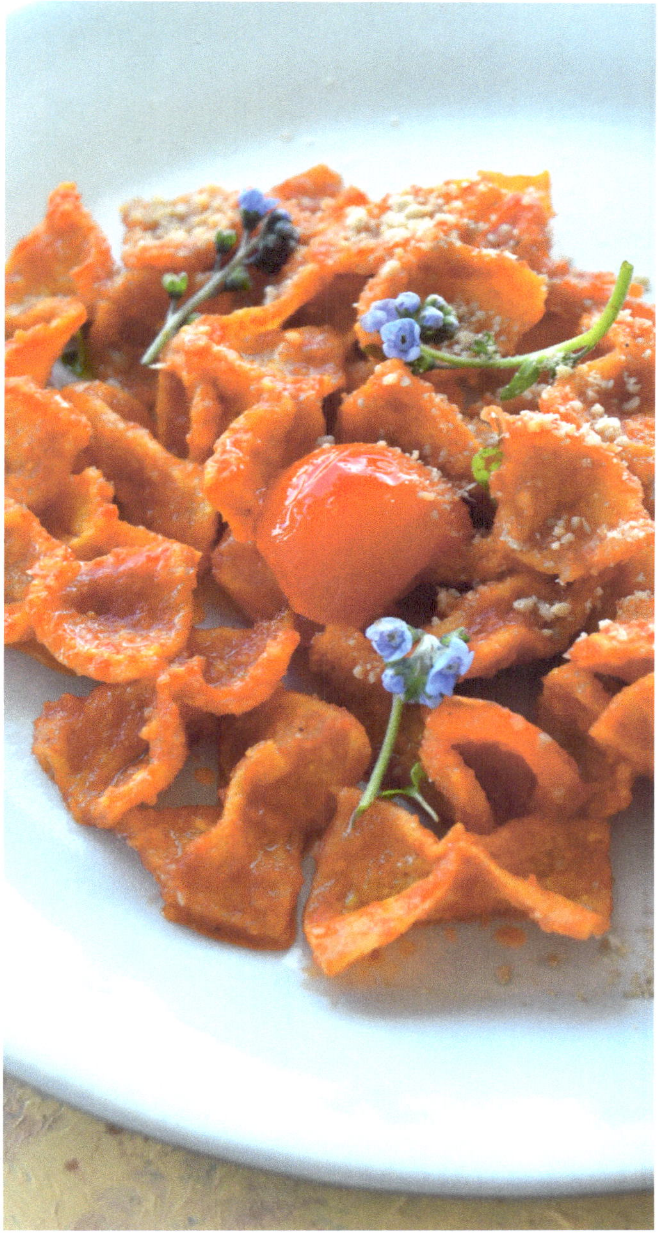

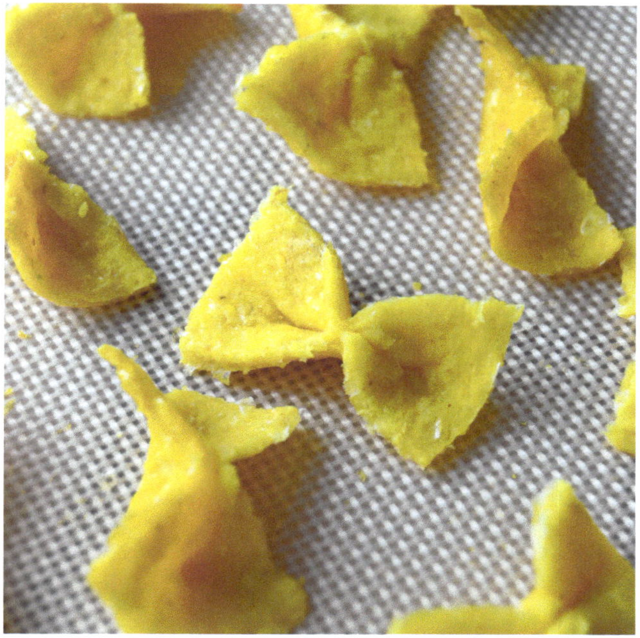

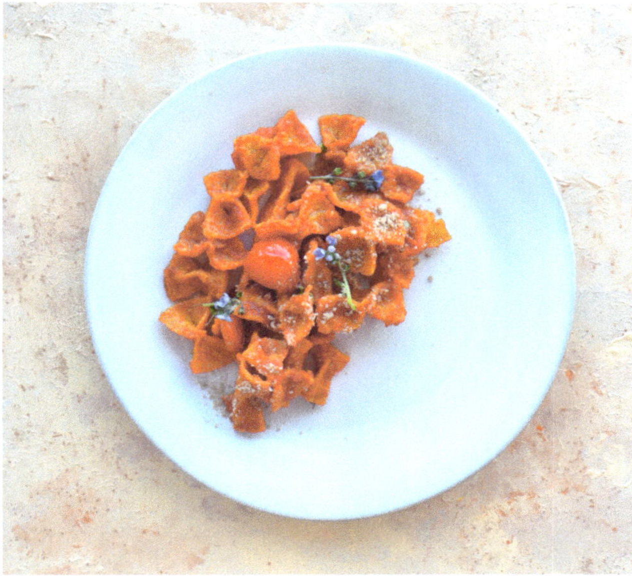

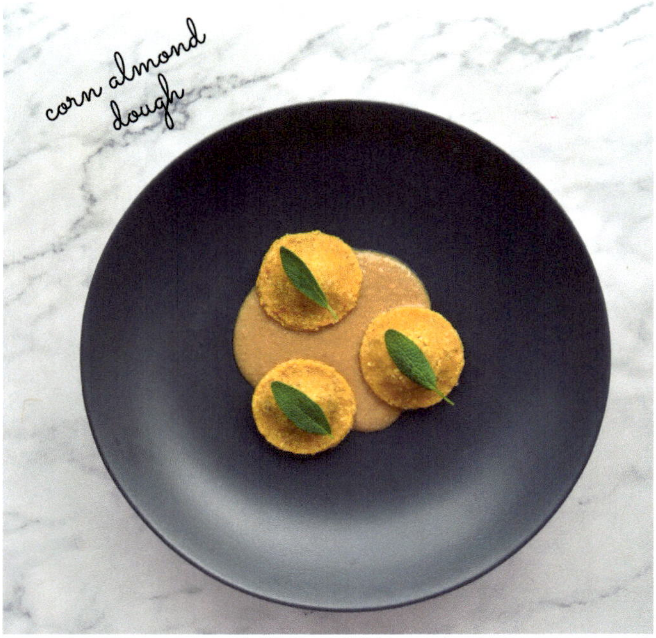
corn almond
dough

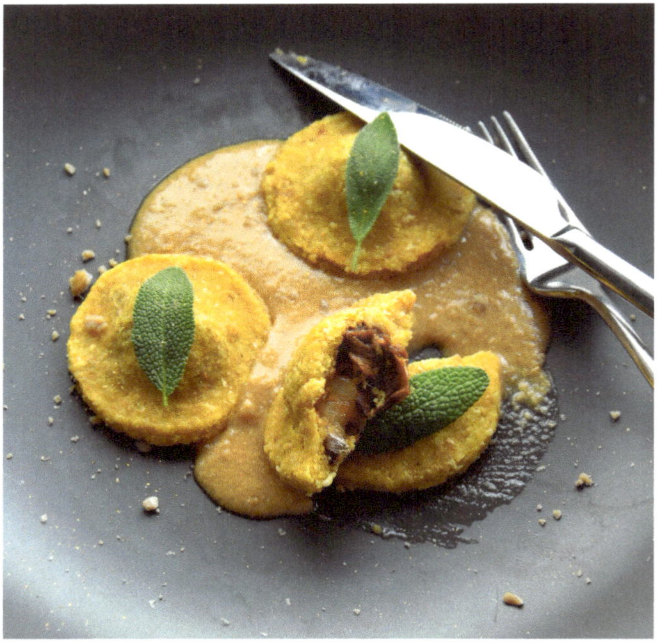

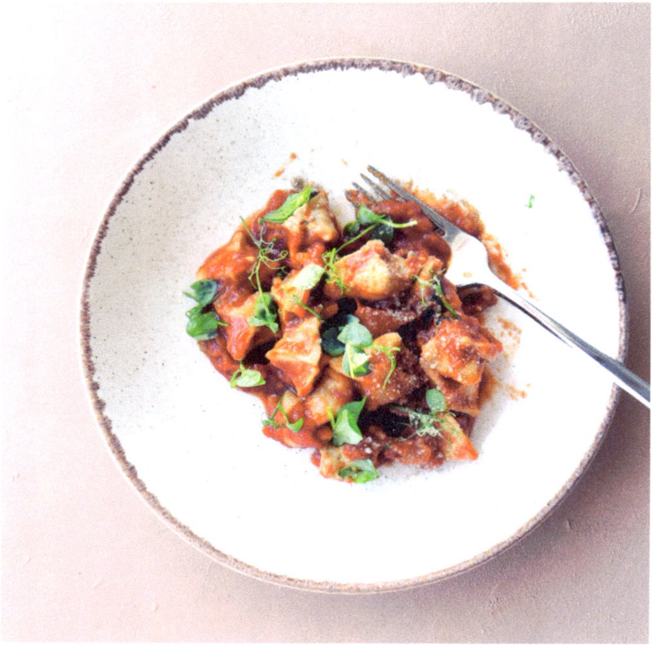

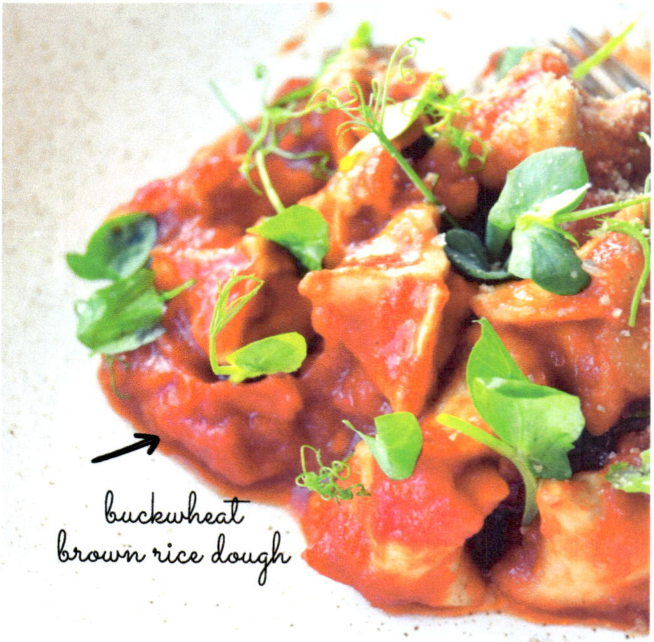
buckwheat
brown rice dough

RAWIOLI TWO WAYS

Category - Dehydrated-Raw
Time - 30 min prep + 2 hrs dehydration
Serves - 4 person

Equipment - Food processor, dehydrator, 2.5-3 cm ring cutter
Personal note - A real chewy pasta feeling!

Corn almond dough ingredients

100 g fresh heirloom corn
1 cup almond flour
1 cup oat flour
1/2 cup water
2 tbsp psyllium husk powder
1 tsp salt

Cream sauce

1 tbsp tahini
1 tbsp coconut aminos or tamari
40 g coconut cream
1 tsp onion powder
1/8 tsp paprika
1/2 tsp mustard powder
1/8 tsp salt

For serving

Pine nuts or rawmesan
Fresh sage
Nutmeg

Alternative dough ingredients (buckwheat & brown rice)

1 cup sprouted buckwheat flour
1/2 cup sprouted brown rice flour
1 tbsp olive oil
1 tbsp psyllium husk powder + 3 tbsp water
120 ml water

Mushroom filling

15 g dried porcini mushrooms
1 celery stalk small diced
2 tbsp chopped walnuts
2 small red pepper chopped
2 pieces sun-dried tomatoes
1 medjool date pitted
1 medium onion thinly sliced
2 tbsp coconut aminos (or 1 tbsp tamari)
1 tsp salt
1 tsp garlic powder
1/4 tsp chili powder
1 tbsp olive oil
1 tbsp lemon juice
Filtered water as needed
1/2 tsp dried oregano
1/8 tsp black pepper

To make ravioli dough

1. Place heirloom fresh corns in a bowl. Cover with warm water. Let it sit for 2-3 hours.
2. Then strain and dry. Transfer corns to a blender.
3. Add 1/2 cup filtered water, salt, almond flour, oat flour and psyllium husk powder.
4. Blend until you get smooth mixture.
5. Once done spread mixture onto the dehydrator trays lined parchment paper.
6. Dehydrate at 42° C for 1-2 hours or until it can be easily flipped.
7. Then transfer the dough onto your cutting board lined parchment paper.

To make alternative ravioli dough

1. If you don't want to use corns, you can also make raw rawioli dough with sprouted whole grain flours. Sprouted buckwheat flour with the starchy sprouted brown rice flour works great. While psyllium gives flexibility, brown rice make your dough softer.
2. Place all ingredients in a mixing bowl except water and oil. Mix well. Then add the water and olive oil. Stir to combine well. Using your hands, knead dough in the bowl, once shaped, remove from the bowl. Dust some buckwheat flour on your working surface. Place the dough and make a ball. Using a rolling pin, roll the dough thinly as much as you can do. Cut the dough into strips and then squares about 4x4 cm.
3. Using a teaspoon, fill each square with mushroom filling. Pinch and close the raviolis.
4. Toss with tomato sauce or your favorite one, place the ravioli in a plate or bowl. 5. Transfer to dehydrator, heat at 42 C for 1-2 hours before serving. Once the ravioli absorb the sauce, it will be softer. As the flours are sprouted and dehydrated, you can also consume the dough without re-dehydration process after combining with the sauce if you like.

To make mushroom filling

1. In a mixing bowl, place porcini mushrooms, sun dried tomatoes and date. Soak in warm water for 5-6 minutes.
2. Then strain and drain. Dice them together. Transfer to a large bowl.
3. Then add the diced celery, bell pepper, and onion. Add the olive oil and mix until the ingredients are well and evenly coated.

3. Spread the mixture on a dehydrator tray lined with paraflexx sheet and dehydrate for 30-45 minutes. This step helps to concentrate the flavours of the vegetables and give a more traditional chilli flavour.
4. Once the vegetables are briefly dehydrated, place them in a bowl and add the chopped walnuts (or pecan, brazil nuts). Set aside while you prepare the sauce.
5. Add the spices to the vegetable mixture and fold together until combined. Taste and adjust the seasonings and texture. Add water to desired consistency, and add coconut aminos (or nama sho-yu, tamari) if you prefer a deeper, more savoury chilli.
6. This mixture tastes best if it is allowed to sit for at least one hour. So it is best to plan ahead and prepare early.

To make cream sauce

1. In a bowl, whisk together all the ingredients until well-combined and emulsified.
2. Taste the sauce; it should strike a balance between umami and tangy creaminess. Adjust the seasonings as needed with salt, pepper, coconut aminos or mustard.
3. Place bowl in the dehydrator. At 42° C, cook the sauce in the dehydrator while assembling the ravioli.

Assembly

1. Drop about 1 to 1 1/2 tbsp of mushroom filling about 4 cm apart all along the dough.
2. When the sheet of dough is fully dotted with dabs of filling mixture, cover filling with other sheet of dough.
3. Using your fingers, gently press dough between each dab of filling to seal it.
4. Cut ravioli into squares with a (zig-zag edged) pastry cutter, or very sharp knife.
5. Allow ravioli to dry for one hour in the dehydrator.
6. Remove sage cream sauce and ravioli from the dehydrator.
7. Place ravioli in a large square bow.
8. Pour the sage cream sauce over the ravioli. Let it heat in the dehydrator for one hour or until soft enough.
9. Serve with pine nuts or rawmesan , fresh sage leaves and a pinch of nutmeg.

Notes: You can also use the corn farfalle pasta dough recipe in this book. It is softer compared this dough recipe.

PEA FARFALLE

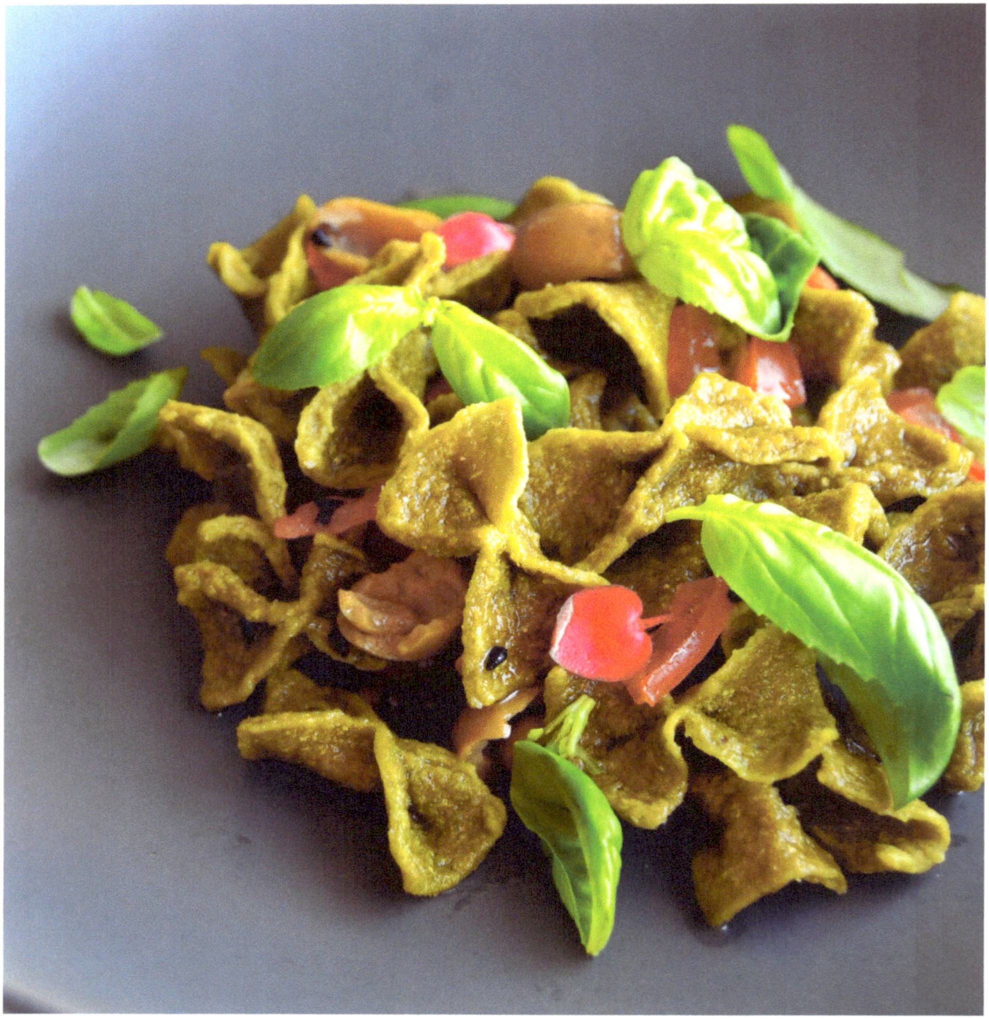

Crafted from 100% organic green peas. You can store in the airtight container up to couple of months... To eat, just soak in warm water for 2-3 minutes. For a true taste of Italy, serve al dente, do not soak too long. Combine with your favorite sauce.

Category - Dehydrated-Raw   Preperation - 20 minutes   Makes - 400 g

Dough ingredients

400 g fresh baby green peas

1 cup water

3 tbsp psyllium husk powder

Instructions

1. Place fresh peas to your blender. Add the water. Blend until smooth.
2. Then add the psyllium husk, blend again till combined.
3. Let it sit for 10 min. until psyllium absorbs the water.
4. When the dough has come together smoothly. If it's feeling moist, add some more psyllium husk into the dough. You want to end up with a ball that's sticky but not too much, it should be still soft.
5. Roll the dough between silicon or parchment paper and roll them out until it is about 1.5mm thick.
(200 g dough per 30x30 cm dehydrator tray)
6. Place dough to your dehydrator sheet lined parchment paper. Dehydrate for 1-2 hours at 42° C until it becomes easily reversible.
7. At this stage you will shape your pasta dough. Cut into desired shape. To make farfalle, take your ravioli wheel cutter and cut the rectangle into strips. Your strips should be approximately 4-5cm wide and 2cm long.
8. Use your thumb and forefinger to pinch the long edges together to form a bow.
9. Repeat with remaining rectangles, then remaining pieces of dough. Arrange the pasta in a single layer on dehydrator sheet. Ensure there is a good amount of space between each shape to avoid them from sticking together.
10. Dehydrate for 4-5 hours or until completely dried.
11. Serve with fresh basil, olive oil, rawmesan or your favorite sauce.

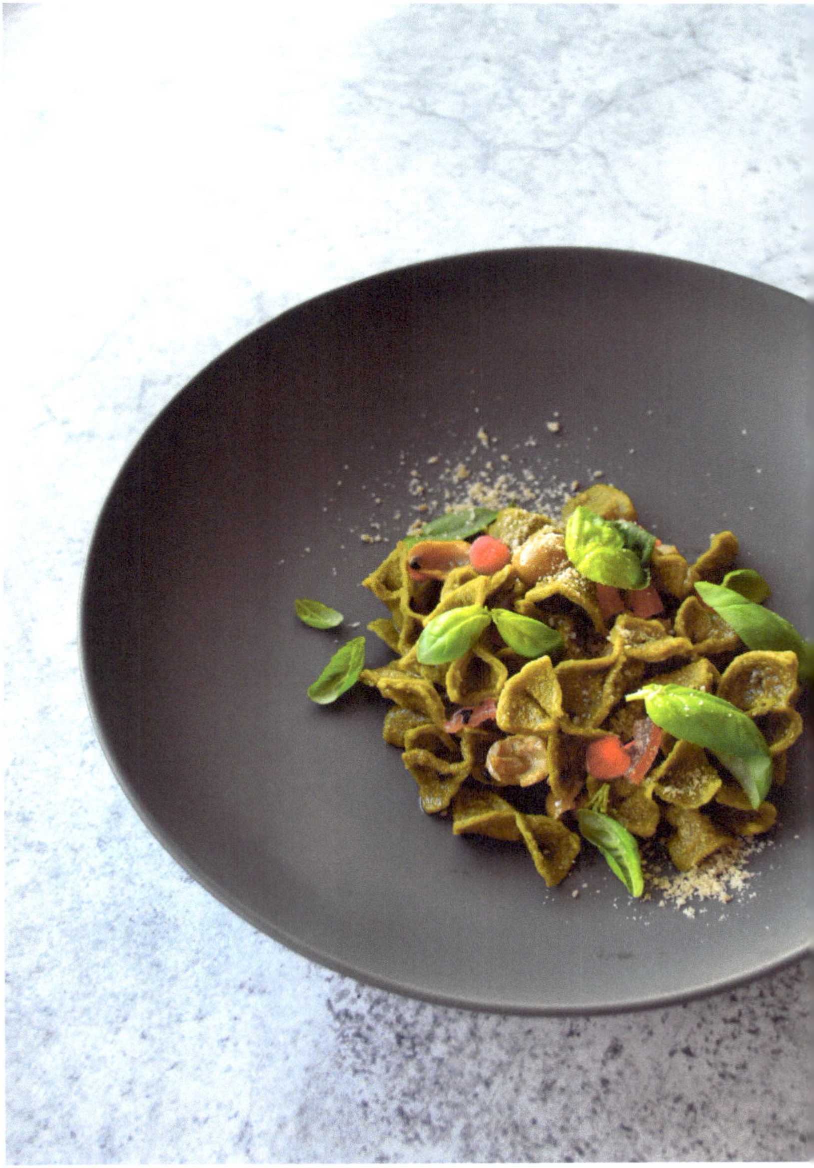

SOUS VIDE CELERIAC

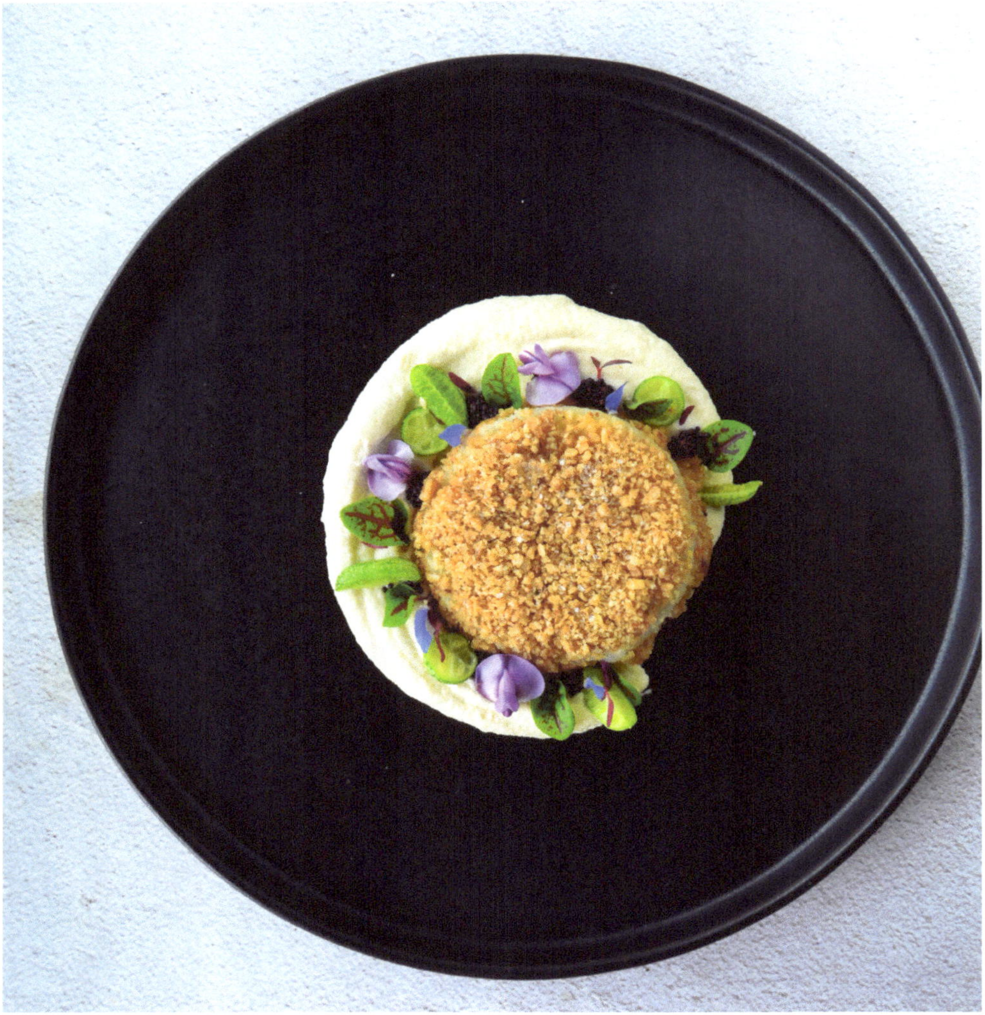

Sous vide technique allows to cook at low temperature of water so there is less risk of over-cooking our fruits & vegetables in the raw food world. Furthermore, sealing your plants before cooking in water helps retain natural plant sugars that would otherwise be diluted in a large volume of cooking water. That means brighter color and fuller flavor, every time.

Category - Sous vide-Raw
Time - 30 min prep + 3 hrs sousvide
Quantity - 2 X 15 cm pizza

Equipment - Food processor, blender, sous vide, 6 cm ring cutter

Ingredients
1 large head celeriac

For the oat crumb
1 cup rolled oats
1/2 tsp salt
1 tsp garlic powder
1 tsp onion powder
1 tbsp lemon zest
2 tbsp nutritional yeast

For the orange cream
1 cup almonds soaked peeled
2 tbsp lemon juice
2 drops doTERRA orange essential oil
1/4 tsp cardamom
1/2 tsp salt
Water as needed

For the garnish
Bean blossoms, vene cress, borage, pepquino, black mustard caviar

Instructions
1. Place celeriac in a large zipper lock or vacuum seal bag. Seal the bag using the water immersion technique or a vacuum sealer on the moist setting. Place the bag in a preheated water bath at 46° C and set the timer for 2-3 hours or until tender.
2. When the timer goes off, remove the bag from the water bath. Transfer the celeriac on your cutting board.
3. Using a round cutter, cut and shape it.

To make oat crumb
1. Place all the ingredients in a food processor.
2. Blend until you get crumb.

To make orange cream
1. Place all the ingredients to a high speed blender.
2. Blender until silky smooth.

Assembly
1. Put the oat crumb into a large bowl.
2. Place the celery ring in the bowl and coat it with the crumb.
3. Take two spoons of orange cream and spread it in a circle in the middle of the plate.
4. Place the oat-covered celery ring over the cream.
5. Pepquino, bean blossom, vene cress, borage, black mustard seeds are recommended as decoration.

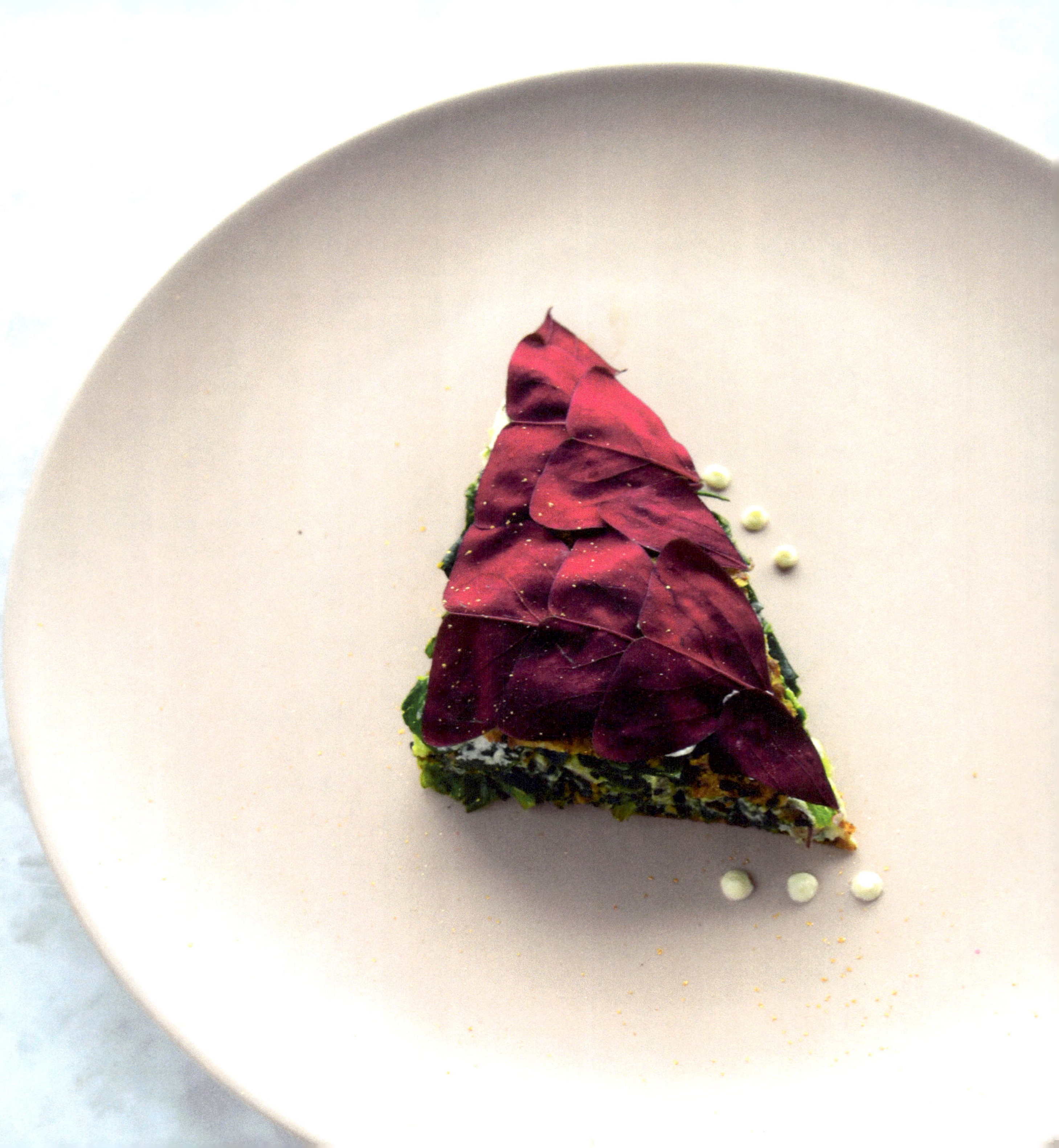

SPINACH BÖREK

Category - Dehydrated- Raw
Preperation - 20 min + 8 hrs dehydration
Quantity - 4-6 person

Equipment - Food processor, dehydrator, piping bag, tea strainer
Personal note - A nostalgic feeling!

Ingredients for the dough*

800 g zucchini peeled
8 tbsp flaxseeds
4 tbsp lemon juice
2 tsp herbs de provence
2 tbsp black sesame seeds to sprinkle
1/2 tsp salt

Plating

Oxalis leaves to decorate
Freeze dried raspberry powder to decorate

Instructions for the dough

1. Peel and wash your zucchini. Cut in four pieces. Add to your food processor. Blend until smooth.
2. To have flax meal, ground flax seeds in a coffee grinder to produce a fine flour.
3. Then add the flax meal, lemon juice and salt to your food processor. Blend until smooth.
4. Pour mixture onto the dehydrator sheets and spread evenly into a circle or square shape. Sprinkle some black sesame over the dough. (I use 30x30 cm dehydrator sheets.)
5. Dehydrate for 6-8 hours at 42° C , or until able to peel off the sheet.
6. Once the nonstick sheets are removed, return to the dehydrator for 1-2 hours, until both sides are dry to the touch but still pliable. Do not dehydrate too long as breaks will occur in the dough. You should obtain a flexible dough and it should be easily rolled up.

* This recipes makes 4 tray dough. If you want to make more, double the ingredients.

spinach börek continued

Hemp cheese cream ingredients

100 g hemp hearts (alternatively sunflower seeds or almonds)
3 tbsp lemon juice
1 stalk leek
1 tsp salt
Water as needed to blend

To make hemp cheese cream

1. Place all ingredients into your blender. Add minimum amount of water as needed to blend.
2. Blend until smooth. Set aside.

Spinach filling ingredients

500 g fresh spinach
3 tbsp olive oil
1 tsp lemon juice
1 tsp salt
1 shallot chopped
1 tsp garlic minced

To make spinach filling

1. Wash and strain your spinach. Finely chop using a sharp knife. Place in a large bowl.
2. Finely chop onion, add over the spinach.
3. Add garlic, lemon juice and olive oil on top.
4. Massage with your hands until wilted well.

Assembly

1. Lay the dough on a work surface. Pour hemp cream in the centre of the dough. Spread through the middle of the dough so that almost reaches the edges.
2. Add the spinach mixture over the hemp cream, spread well.
3. Add another dough sheet on the mixture.
4. Spread hemp cream and spinach again.
5. Repeat the process one more time. Cut in squares or triangle.
6. Decorate with purple oxalis leaves and using a tea strainer sprinkle some freeze dried berry powder and pipe hemp cream dots around the börek. Serve!

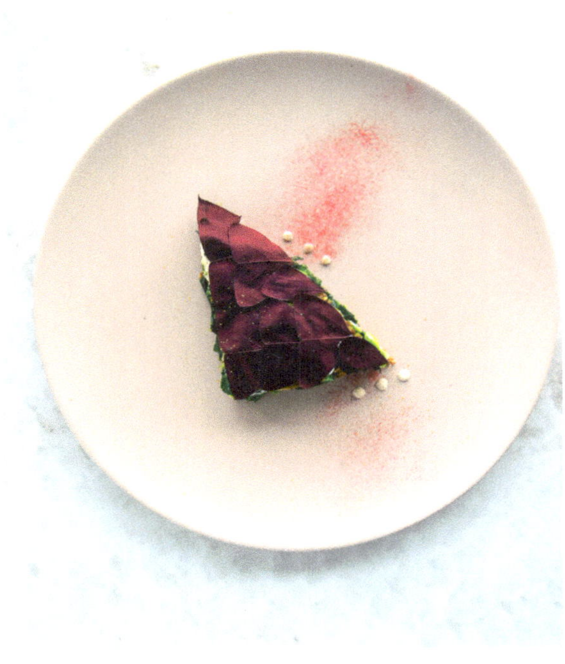

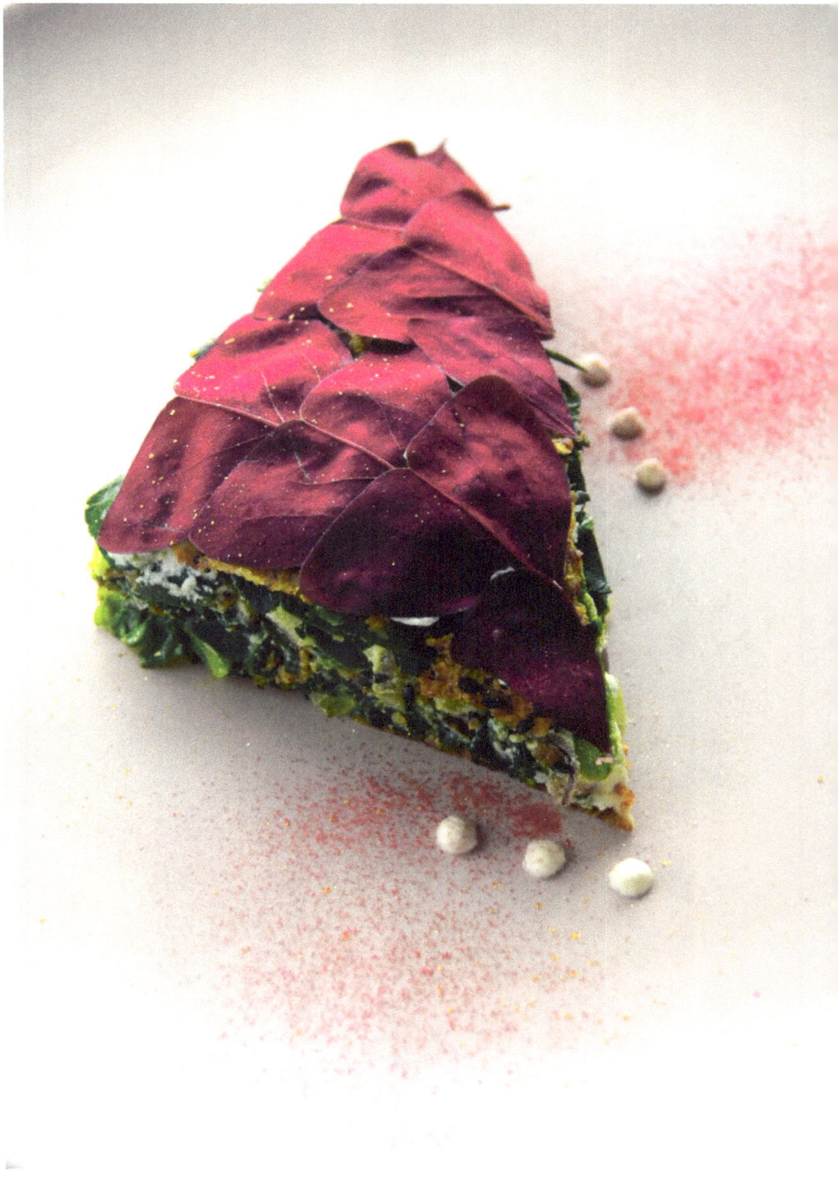

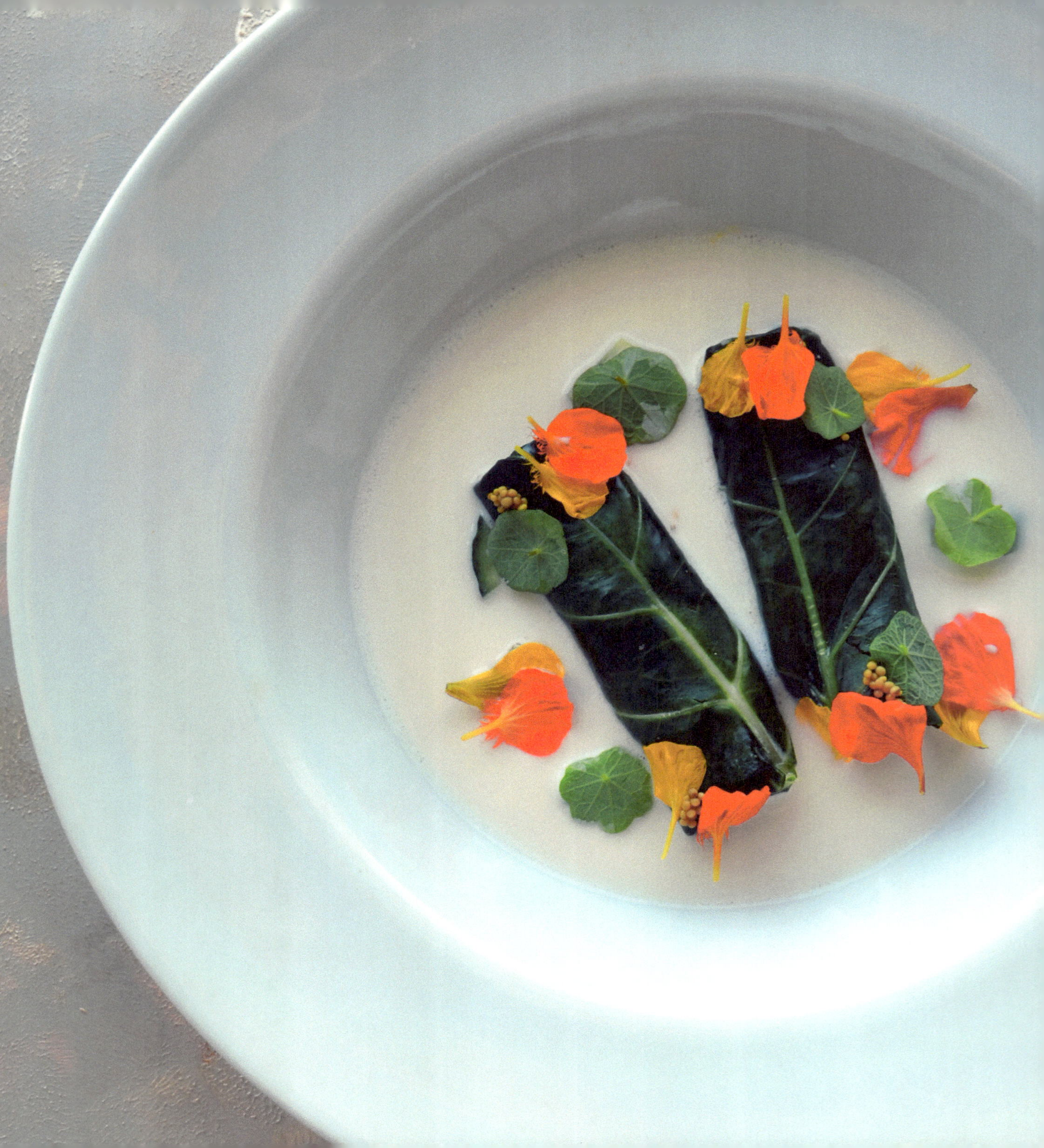

OAT FILLED COLLARD SARMA

Category - Pure-Raw +Dehydrated-Raw
Time - 30 min prep + 3 hrs dehydration
Quantity - 2-4 person

Equipment - food processor, dehydrator
Note - sarma is a similar to dolmas. Dolma means "stuffed veggies" and sarma means ""wrapped leaves" in Turkish.

Ingredients

200 g fresh wine leaves or collard greens
1 cup gf sprouted rolled oats
1 cup water
1 large onion thinly sliced
1 tsp olive oil
1 tbsp maple syrup
25 g pine nuts
40 g dried blackcurrants
3-4 cherry tomatoes cut into small pieces
1/2 tsp all spice
1/2 tsp cinnamon powder
1/2 tsp peppermint
1/2 tsp salt or more if you need

Instructions

1. Thinly slice onion, massage well with olive oil. Place on the dehydrator tray lined silicon paper. Dehydrate for 2-3 hours at 42° C until caramelized.
2. Then chop onions into small pieces, set aside.
3. Place gluten free rolled oats in a bowl, cover with 1 cup warm water. Let it sit for 1-2 hours until the oats absorb the all water and get soften. If they are still juicy, using a sieve, strain the excess water. Put back oats into bowl.
4. In a small bowl, place dried blackcurrants, cover with warm water. Let it sit for 15 minutes. Once soften, strain the excess water.
5. Add the onions, maple, pine nuts, black currants, cinnamon, all spice, peppermint and salt into your oat bowl. Cut tomatoes in small cubes. Add to your bowl.
6. Using a fork or spoon, give it a good toss until well combined.
7. Carefully separate out a grape/collard leaf from the batch. Wash your leaves, place in a large bowl. Add warm water at maximum 42° C, let them soak for 30 minutes. Cut away the stems. Once soften enough, they are ready to roll.

sarma continued

8. Place your grape/collard leaf shiny side down so that the leaf veins are facing up. The veins will be on the inside of the roll and make for a neater appearance. Place your filling in the center of the leaf, near the bottom. you will find 1 tablespoon to be a good start for filling amount. Use less for smaller leaves.
9. Then, fold up the bottom left and right sides at a bit of an angle. You want to cover the filling and try to start "squaring off" the leaf.
10. Now, take the part with the filling and roll it over itself going toward the top of the leaf.
11. Next, fold in the sides. This can just be done at a straight angle. You want to enclose the filling so it doesn't fall out either end.
12. Roll the rest of it up toward the top. Make sure you don't overstuff the sarma or roll it too tightly.

Tips:

Always try to start with larger grape leaves without holes or tears. This will help you practice and as you become more proficient, you can move on to the trickier leaves.

Almond foam (optional)
150 ml almond milk
1 tsp soy or sunflower lecithin powder
1 tsp coconut milk

To make almond foam
1. Place almond milk in the blender. Sift on the sugar and lecithin. Blend well.
2. Using the immersion blender, blend the liquid until it creates a large amount of foam. This process can take anywhere from 60 seconds up to a few minutes. Let the foam stabilize for a minute and then you can use it.

Toppings
Nasturtium Flowers
Pickled mustard (optional)

Assembly
1. Place sarmas into a plate.
2. Pour the foam in the plate.
3. Decorate with nasturtiums.

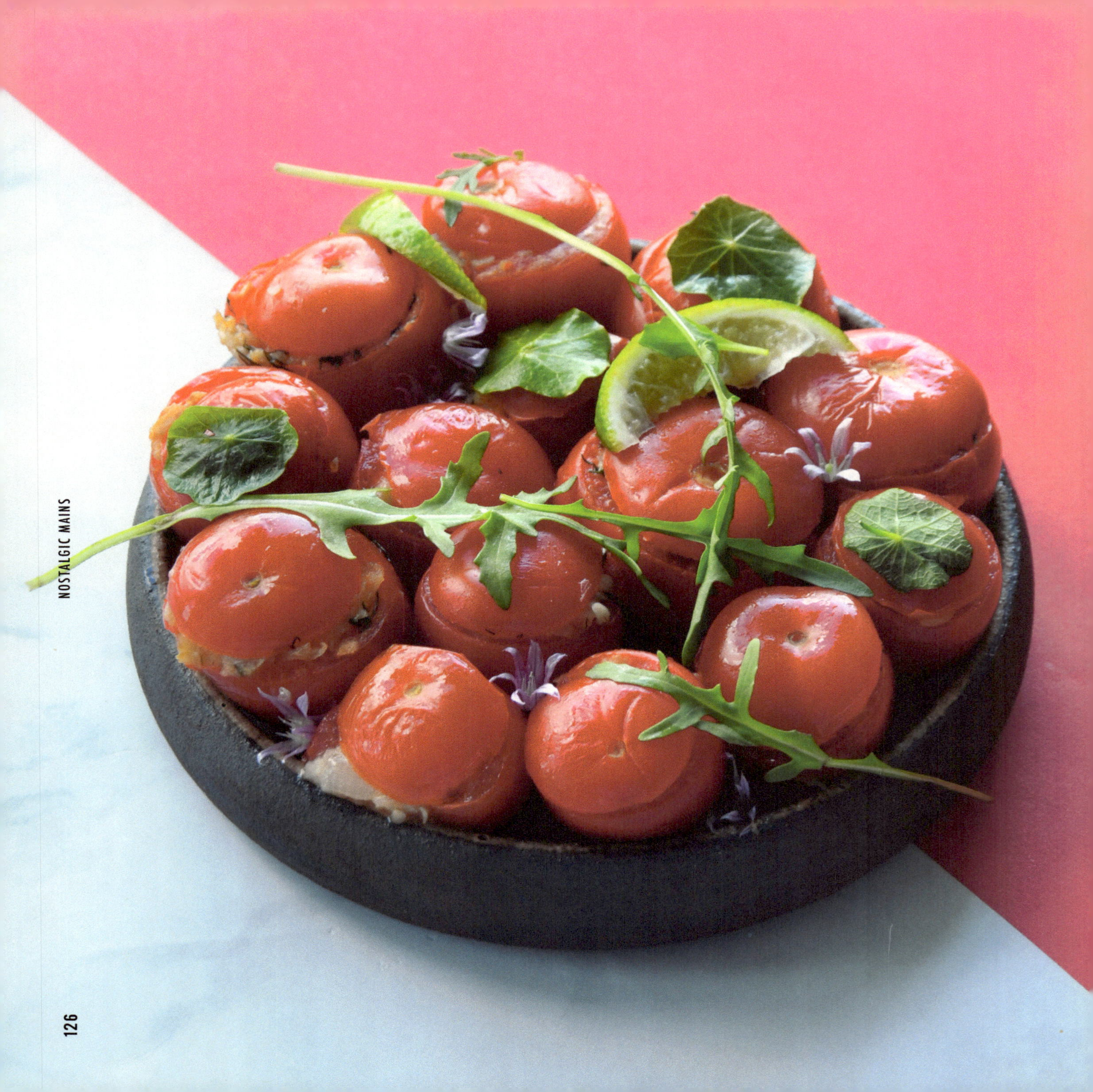

GREEK STYLE STUFFED TOMATO DOLMAS

Category - Dehydrated OR Pure Raw
Time - 30 min prep + 3 hrs dehydration
Quantity - 4-6 person
Equipment - Dehydrator
Note - A satisfying raw eating experience

Ingredients

1 kg cherry tomatoes
1 large medium onion
1 cup gf sprouted rolled oats
Juice of 2 lemon
1/2 bunch fresh dill
1/2 tsp salt
2 tbsp olive oil
Garden rockets and nasturtium to serve
Lemon wedges to serve

Instructions

1. Slice almost through the stem end of each tomato, but do not sever as it will serve as a cover. Scoop out inside of each tomato with a teaspoon. Save pulp from 4 tomatoes and set aside. (You can use the remaining pulp in place of diced tomatoes in another recipe. It freezes well).
2. Thinly slice onion, massage well with olive oil. Place on the dehydrator tray lined silicon paper. Dehydrate for 2-3 hours at 42° C until caramelized.
3. Then chop onions into small pieces, set aside.
4. Place gluten free sprouted rolled oats in a bowl, cover with 1 cup warm water. Let it sit for 1-2 hours until the oats absorb the all water and get soften. If they are still juicy, using a sieve, strain the excess water. Put back oats into bowl.
5. Once soften, strain the excess water. Add the onions, lemon juice, salt and dill, mix well.
6. Spoon the oat mixture among tomato shells and top with the reserved tops.
7. Dehydrate at 42° C for 3-4 hours and arrange the tomato dolmas on a serving platter and serve. They also can be eaten without dehydration process, will be still delicious! Serve with arugula, nasturtium, chive blossoms and lemon wedges if you like.

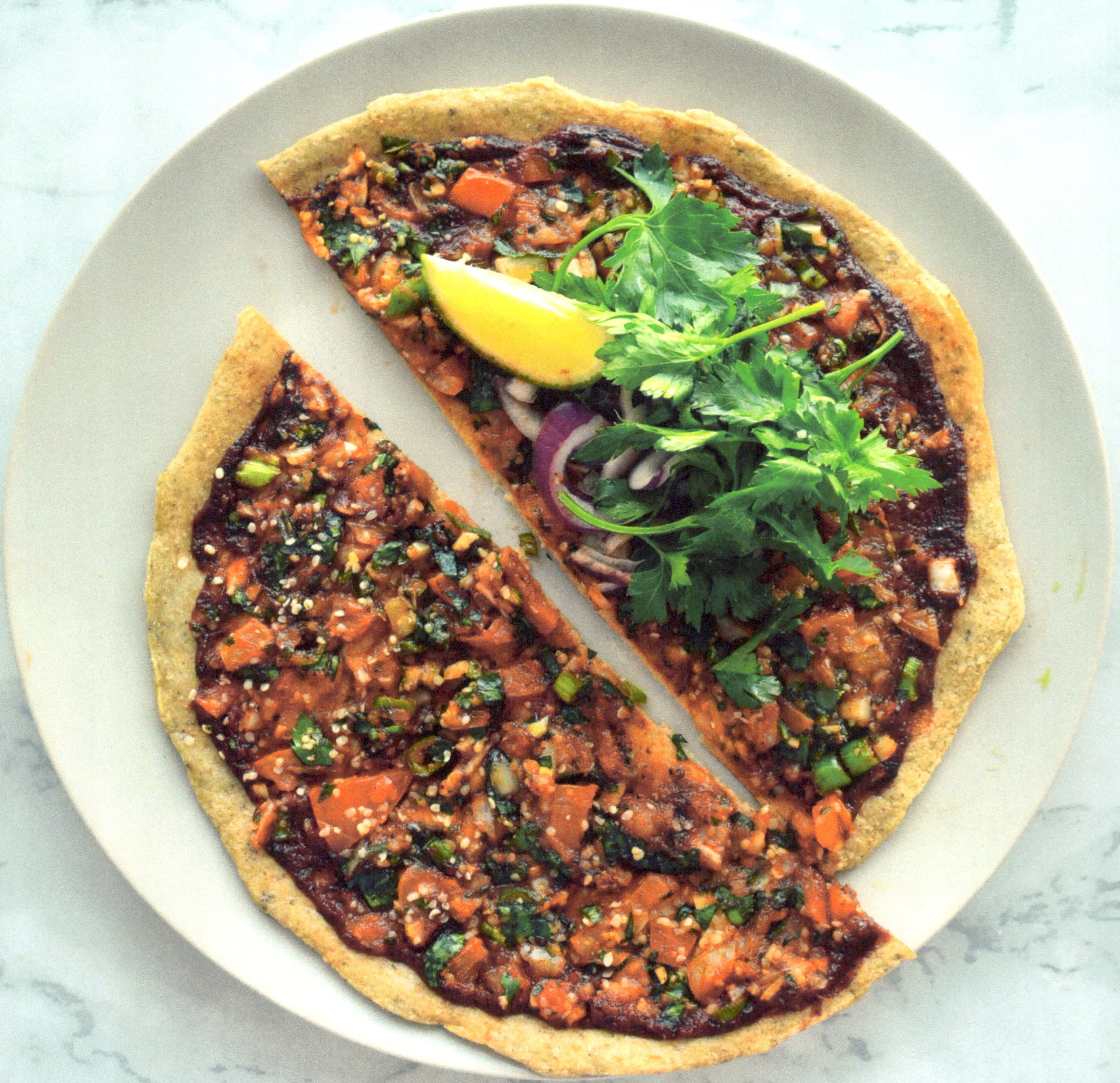

TURKISH RAWMACUN

Category - Dehydrated-Raw
Time - 20 min prep + 8 hrs dehydration
Quantity - 2 X 30 cm lahmacun or 3 x 20cm

Equipment - Food processor, dehydrator
Raw version of turkish lahmacun, a.k.a cheeseless turkish pizza

Crust ingredients

1 large kohlrabi (250g measured after peeled)
55 g sprouted buckwheat flour
2 tbsp sesame oil
1/4 cup psyllium husk powder
1 cup water
1 tsp salt

Dende oil (optional)

1/4 cup coconut oil
1/8 tsp cayenne
1 whole chili
1/4 tsp salt

Toppings

1 medium yellow onion, finely grated
3 to 4 cloves garlic, finely grated
1 cup finely chopped parsley leaves
2 medium ripe tomatoes, finely grated
1/2 medium green pepper, finely grated
1 tbsp red pepper puree
1 tbsp sun-dried tomato puree
1 tbsp red pepper flakes
1 tbsp sumac
1 tbsp hemp hearts (optional)
1 tsp salt
lemon wedges, for garnish

rawmacun continued

To make crust

1. Peel your kohlrabi, cut into small pieces. Place into a high speed blender.
2. Add water and sesame oil. Blend until smooth puree.
3. Then add the sprouted buckwheat flour, salt and psyllium husk, blend until well combined. Let it sit for 30 seconds.
4. Then immediately pour onto the dehydrator sheets lined silicon paper.
5. Using a silicon spatula, spread mixture in a circle.
6. Dehydrate at 42° C. This kohlrabi crust does not require very long hours of baking. the dough will become pliable in 1-1.5 hours. Then carefully remove it from the ends and flip it over and bake another 1-2 hours.

To make topping mixture

1. Process the peppers, onion, tomato, garlic, and parsley in your food processor in batches according to its size.
2. Once the veggies are finely pureed, transfer them to a fine mesh sieve placed over a bowl.
3. Lightly strain the veggie mixture of excess juices. (Reserve the juices for later.)
4. Place the vegetable puree in a large bowl along with olive oil, red pepper and tomato paste (to make these, simply blend red pepper and sun dried tomatoes with little water in the blender and then squeeze the excess water using a strainer), red pepper flakes (according to your heat preference), salt, and pepper.
5. Mix well until a soft paste forms. (If the mixture looks dry, add a splash of the reserved vegetable juices to the mixture.)
6. Cover the mixture and let the flavors develop for 30 minutes.

To make dende oil

1. Blend all the dende oil ingredients in blender until smooth.
2. Pour through a strainer with a coffee filter inside. Let drain the mixture.
3. Store in sealed container or bottle in refrigerator up to a week. Keep at room temperature before using or let it sit near to dehydrator to get a liquid mixture before using. Then shake and use.

Assembly

1. Once both sides of the dough are cooked, lightly oil the outer edge of the crust with olive oil. Remove silicon sheet and place dough on the dehydrator tray.
2. Spread the topping thinly and evenly over the top of each dough round with your fingers. Don't press down too hard.
3. Place in the dehydrator, bake at 42° C for 3-4 hours or until desired cooked consistency.
4. Drizzle dende oil onto the lahmacun. Serve the lahmacuns with lemon wedges for squeezing and a plate of sliced onions mixed with sumac and sprigs of parsley.

This recipe is designed for immediate consumption! It is best when consumed as baked. If will eat later, then dehydrate until warm.

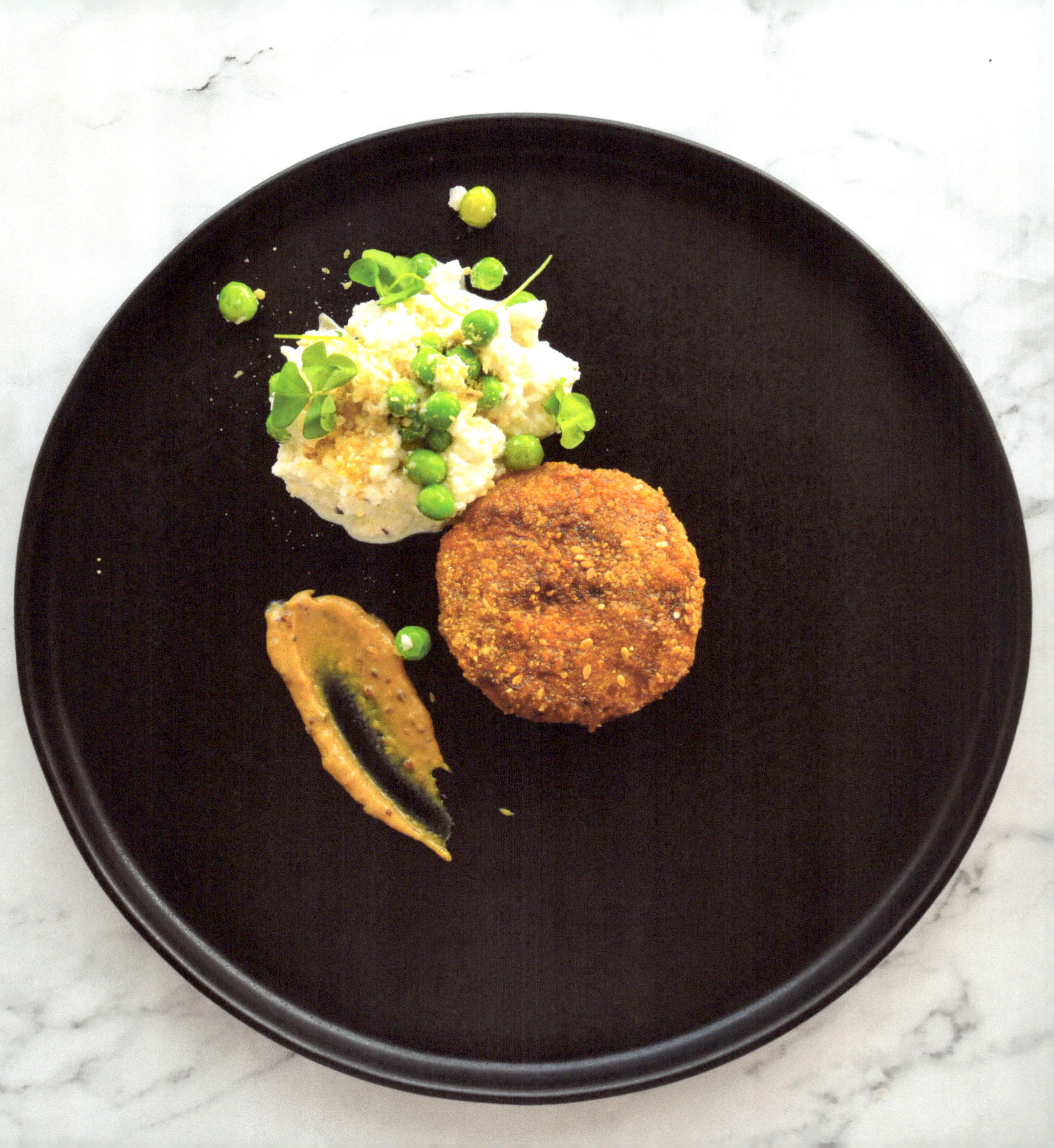

KOHLRAWI SCHNITZEL WITH CREAMY PEA RISOTTO

Category - Sous Vide + Dehydrated-Raw
Time - 30 min prep + 2-3 hrs dehydration
Quantity - 2 person

Equipment - Blender, non-stick sheets, sous vide, spatula, 5cm ring cutter, dehydrator

Ingredients

1 large kohlrabi
1 tbsp olive oil
150 ml water
1 tbsp coconut aminos
1 tbsp maple syrup
1 tbsp nutritional yeast

Batter

1/3 cup oat flour
1/2 cup plant milk

Crumb

1/3 cup buckini
1/2 tsp salt
1/4 tsp paprika powder
1/2 tsp turmeric powder
1 tsp sesame seeds

Instructions

1. Take any additional leaves off the kohlrabi and wash it.
2. Cut the kohlrabi in 4-6 slices (about 8mm) and around the slices with a veggie peeler to remove the outer layer.
3. Drop the slices into a bowl of iced water as soon as they are cut.
4. When you have finished cutting the kohlrabi, remove one slice from the iced water.
5. Punch out a circle using round cutter 5cm in diameter, then return the circle to the water.
6. Discard the rest of the slice and repeat with the remaining slices. Store in the water until needed.
7. Mix together the water, coconut aminos, maple and nutritional yeast in a bowl.
8. Take the sliced kohlrabi out of the iced water, place them in a vacuum bag and pour over the liquid. Using a chamber sealer set on full pressure, seal the bag until the kohlrabi is fully compressed. Chill the bag in the fridge for 1 hour.

kohlrabi schnitzel continued

9. While the kohlrabi is being marinated in the fridge, prepare the batter and crumble for the coating.
10. After 2 hours, place the bag in the water bath and leave to cook at 42° C for 3-4 hours or until cooked well.
11. Once cooked, remove the kohlrabi slices from the vacuum bag and drain off the liquid.

Assembly:

1. Prepare three shallow plates for breading: one plate with plant-based milk, one with oat flour, and one with buckini crumb mixture (mix all the crumb ingredients in a bowl).
2. Dredge kohlrabi slices in oat flour first, then transfer them to plant-based milk, and toss them in the buckini crumb mixture until they are covered all over.
3. To get an even thicker breading, dip them once more in plant-based milk, then cover them with buckini crumb for a second time.
4. Let them dehydrate on 42° C heat for about 1-2 hour per side until form well and stick to the slices.
5. Serve with salad, dijon mustard and lemon or in a bun with thinly sliced fresh red onion, tomatoes, greens and your favorite sauce.

CREAMY RISOTTO WITH PEAS

Category - Pure-Raw
Time - 30 min prep

Equipment - Blender
Quantity - 2 person

Ingredients
240 g cauliflower
1/2 cup fresh green peas
Fresh dill
Rawmesan (mixture of sunflower seeds, nutritional yeast, salt and garlic powder)

Cream
1 cup raw almonds or cashews soaked
2 tbsp nutritional yeast
1 tsp apple cider vinegar
1 tbsp olive oil (add +1 tbsp if you go with the almonds)
1/2 tsp salt or miso
Blackpepper to taste
1/4 cup water or more as you need

Instructions
1. Wash and cut your cauliflower into chunks, place into food processor. Blend well until you get rice-like form.
2. Then transfer it to a sieve, using a spoon press well and remove the excess water of cauliflower rice.
3. Transfer cauliflower-rice to a large bowl.
4. Soak cashews or almonds overnight or for 4-5 hours. Drain and rinse well.
5. Place into a high speed blender.
6. Add the rest of the ingredients. Just add minimum amount of water to blend, no more. If you are using almonds, you may need to add some olive oil.
7. Once done, mix the cauliflower-rice with the sauce. Toss well until well combined.
8. Add the green peas and toss well.
9. Serve with fresh dill and rawmesan if desired.

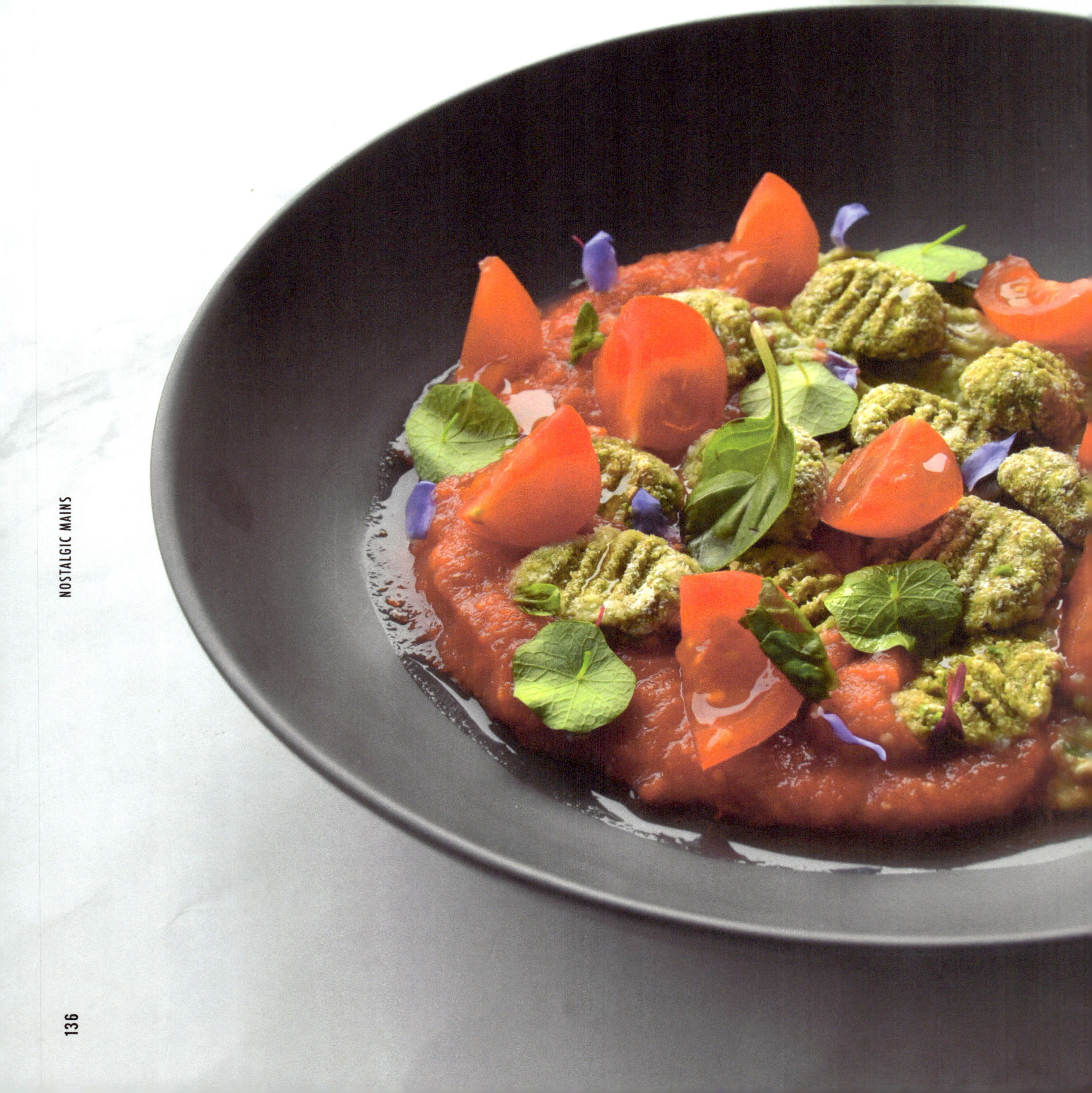

GNOCCHI WITH BASIL PESTO

Category - Dehydrated-Raw
Time - 30 min prep + 3 hrs dehydration
Quantity - 3-4 person

Equipment - Food processor, dehydrator
Perfectly pillowy pasta dumplings

Dough ingredients

3 zucchinis (280g measured after peeled)
1/2 cup green peas (70g)
5 tbsp psyllium husk powder
5 tbsp buckwheat flour
1 tbsp coconut flour
1 tsp garlic powder
1 tsp onion powder
1/4 tsp blackpepper
1/4 tsp salt

Instructions

1. Place raw buckwheats in a bowl, cover with water. Let it sit for 2 hours, then wash, rinse and dry. Place on the dehydrator tray lined silicon sheet. Dehydrate for 4 hours at 42° C or until completely dried. Then transfer to a high speed blender, make it flour.
2. Chop the peeled zucchinis and throw them in to a food processor, add the peas, buckwheat flour, coconut flour, psyllium husk, garlic, onion powder, pepper, and salt. Blend until well combined. Raw food recipes work different for everyone depends on how watery zucchinis are, so feel free to add more buckwheat flour and psyllium husk if the mixture is too wet.
3. Roll small dough pieces with your hands and form them into small pasta pillows, in a rounded rectangle shape. Spread out each gnocchi pasta piece on a silicon sheets upon a dehydrator tray.
4. Using a fork, press the prongs of the fork gently onto the top of each gnocchi piece, leaving the lines pressed into the dough.
5. Dehydrate at 42° C for 2-3 hours.

Pesto Sauce

1/2 bunch basil

1/2 avocado

1 tsp minced garlic

2 tbsp pine nuts or walnut

Juice of 1/2 lemon

Salt to taste

Tomato Sauce

300 g cherry tomatoes

3 slices of sun dried tomatoes

2 dates

1/2 mexican pepper

1/4 tsp salt

Halved cherry tomatoes to serve

Fresh basil and borage to garnish

Instructions

1. To make pesto sauce, wash and drain your basil, peel your avocado, cut tomatoes in two.
2. Throw all the ingredients into a blender, blend until smooth or leave it slightly chunky if you like.
3. To make tomato sauces, place sun dried tomatoes in warm water for 5 minutes, then transfer to a high speed blender, add all the tomato sauce ingredients. Blend until smooth and thick. Let it sit in dehydrator for 1-2 hours if you want warm.

Assembly

1. Place your dehydrated gnocchi in a bowl.
2. Pour the pesto and tomato sauce over the gnocchi. Stir well. Alternatively you can serve sauces on the left of your gnocchi.
3. Add extra halved cherry tomatoes, basil, borage along with black pepper and salt.
4. Serve warm.

OYSTER-LIKE NORDIC SUSHI

Category - Sous Vide + Pure-Raw
Time - 20 minutes
Quantity- 2-4 person

Equipment - Sous vide, bamboo sushi mat, peeler, cling film, a freshly sharpened chef's knife.
Personal note - The most important aspect of this dish – the flavor. Tomatoes do naturally contain a very high umami profile just as tuna does, but it still needs some marinade of some sort to give it a slight ocean-like taste.

Rice ingredients

1 cup gf sprouted nordic oats
1 small red onion diced
1 tbsp unroasted sesame oil
1/2 cup warm water
4-5 tbsp lemon juice
2 tbsp fresh dill chopped
1/2 tsp salt
1 tbsp psyllium husk powder

Other components

Chive blossoms for garnish
Lingonberry jam (page 143)
1 thinly sliced avocado to roll
Freshly squeezed lemon juice to serve

Sous Vide Tomato Filling

3 pieces heirloom tomatoes or (thinly sliced green papayas)
1 tbsp coconut aminos or tamari
1 tbsp olive oil
1/4 tsp salt
1 cup water
1 tsp seaweed blend (from Lofoten Seaweed)

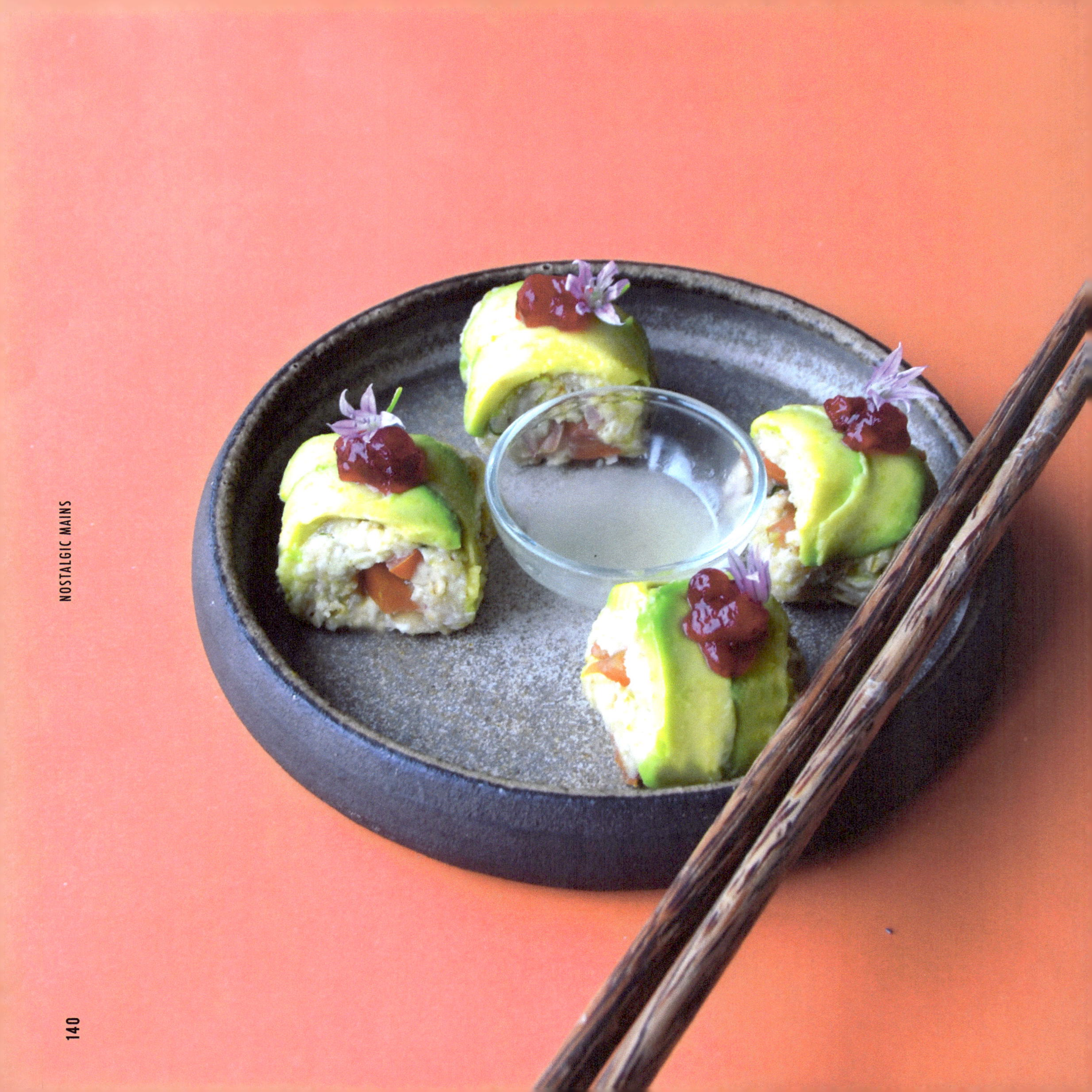

Instructions

For the sous vide tomatoes

1. To make reduction, combine seaweed blend, water, coconut aminos, and salt in a bowl.
2. Drop the tomatoes in warm water for 15 minutes to 20.
3. Then transfer the tomatoes in an ice bath.
4. The skins should come off easily by now. Peel, discard the seeds and cut each tomato into quarters.
5. Put the tomatoes in the seaweed stock and leave to marinate for at least 6 hours. Overnight would certainly make them more flavorful.
6. Put the tomatoes with the marinade in a sous vide bag, cook for 6 hours at 46° C.

For the oat rice

1. Place oats in a bowl, cover with warm water, let it sit for 30 minutes until the oats absorb all the water. Then rinse in cold water.
2. Then add the rest of the ingredients, stir well using a spoon. Let it sit for 5 minutes until psyllium absorbs all the water content.

Assembly

1. Place a cling film on a bamboo mat, then place thinly sliced avocados on the cling film.
2. Place the oat rice on the avocado slices, smooth with the help of a paddle.
3. Layer tomatoes on the oat rice, and roll it up tightly. Slice with a sharp knife, place 1 tsp lingon jam on the top of sushi, garnish with chive blossoms and serve with lemon juice. Let it sit in the refrigerator at least 3 hours before serving.

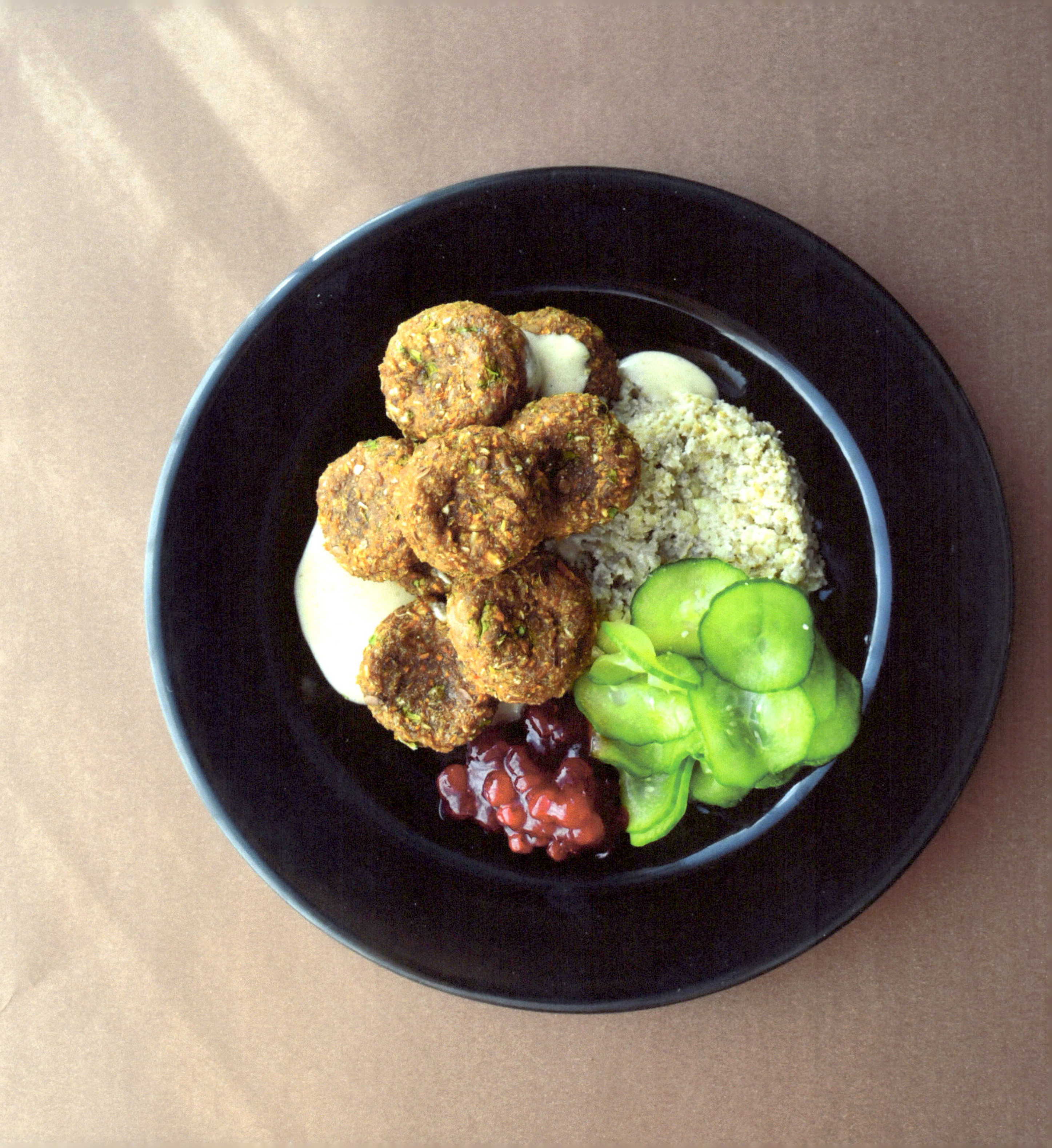

SWEDISH MEATBALLS

Category - Dehydrated-Raw

Time - 40 min prep + 5 hrs dehydration

Equipment - Food processor, dehydrator

Quantity - 4-6 person

Personal note - NUT-FREE

Meatball ingredients

1 cup sprouted rolled oats

1 cup water

1/4 cup fresh green peas

1 small carrot

1 white onion

15g dried porcini

1 tbsp coconut aminos or tamari

1 tbsp flaxseeds

2 tbsp psyllium husk powder

Handful fresh parsley

1/4 tsp black pepper

1/2 tsp salt

1/2 tsp ground nutmeg

Mashed Parsnip

1 cup parsnip

1/4 cup sunflower seeds

1 tbsp maple

1/2 tsp turmeric powder

1 clove garlic minced

1 tbsp lemon juice

1/2 tsp thyme and rosemary blend

1 tbsp olive oil

1/2 tsp salt

Gravy Sauce

1 cup coconut cream

1 tbsp coconut aminos or tamari

1 tbsp olive oil

1 tsp garlic powder

1 tsp onion powder

1 tbsp dried shiitake powder

1/2 tsp dried thyme and rosemary blend

1/4 tsp black pepper

1/2 tsp salt

Pickled Cucumber

1 large english cucumber thinly sliced

1 tbsp maple syrup

1 1/2 tsp salt

1/2 cup apple cider vinegar

1/2 cup water

Lingonberry Jam

300g fresh lingonberries

150g coconut sugar

Instructions

Pickled cucumber

1. In a small to medium bowl, combine the salt, maple, cider vinegar and water. Stir until the maple and salt are completely dissolved.
2. Add the thinly sliced cucumbers.
3. Use the back of a spoon to adjust the cucumbers so they are submerged in the brine. Let the cucumbers soak for about an hour, then they're ready to use.
4. Store in a tight fitting container, with the cucumbers covered in the brining liquid.

Mashed parsnip

1. Blend all the ingredients together in a food processor, for a good few minutes, until the texture is creamy and resembles mashed parsnip.
2. You may need to add a tablespoon of water to help with the blending process. Don't add more than one or two, as it will end up too watery.
3. Serve immediately or set aside at room temperature. If refrigerated, you may want to warm up your mashed parsnips slightly in the dehydrator before serving.

Lingonberry jam

1. Place lingonberries in a jar. Add 50% by weight of powdered coconut sugar. (Grind coconut sugar before).
2. Stir or shake every now and again until the coconut sugar has all dissolved, which might take a day or more. Have a taste and add a little more sugar if desired, but avoid adding so much sugar that it will not dissolve. (Some people squash some of the berries with the back of a spoon to release some of their juice to make it easier to dissolve the sugar, but I try and avoid doing this as I prefer the berries to be left whole.)
3. Store in a cool dark place in sterilised jars.

Meatballs

1. Place dried porcini in a bowl, cover with warm water, let it sit for 10 minutes then strain and dry.
2. Place oats in a bowl, add 1 cup water. Let it sit for 30 minutes. Then transfer to your food processor.
3. Add the porcini mushrooms, peas, carrot and onion. Process until well combined.
4. Add the rest of the ingredients. Blend until you get dough-like texture.
5. Take a heaped teaspoon of the mixture and roll into a ball in your hands. Place on a plate and repeat until all the mixture has gone. It should make about 15-20 balls. Don't make them too big.
6. Dehydrate meatballs in the dehydrator at 42° C for 5-6 hours or until desired crispy consistency.

Gravy sauce

1. Place all gravy sauce ingredients in a blender.
2. Blend until well combined and thick.

Assembly

1. Place mashed parsnip into your place, add meatballs.
2. Pour gravy sauce over the meatballs.
3. Serve with lingonberry jam and pickled cucumber.

Notes: If don't have fresh lingonberries where you live in, use raspberries, cherries, blackberries or blueberries.

timeless sweets

Deconstructed trend taking over the dessert scene!

By dividing traditional desserts into their delicious components, we have created a whole new tasted experience that takes a familiar flavor and turns it on its head. Undressed, uncooked, undone and undeniably delectable, these deconstructed sweets are a point of culinary controversy among the foodies of the world. The ingredients are all there, but presented in an entirely different way. Even if you are sure of what to eat, these delightful deconstructions make some damn good deviations from the dishes we all know and love!

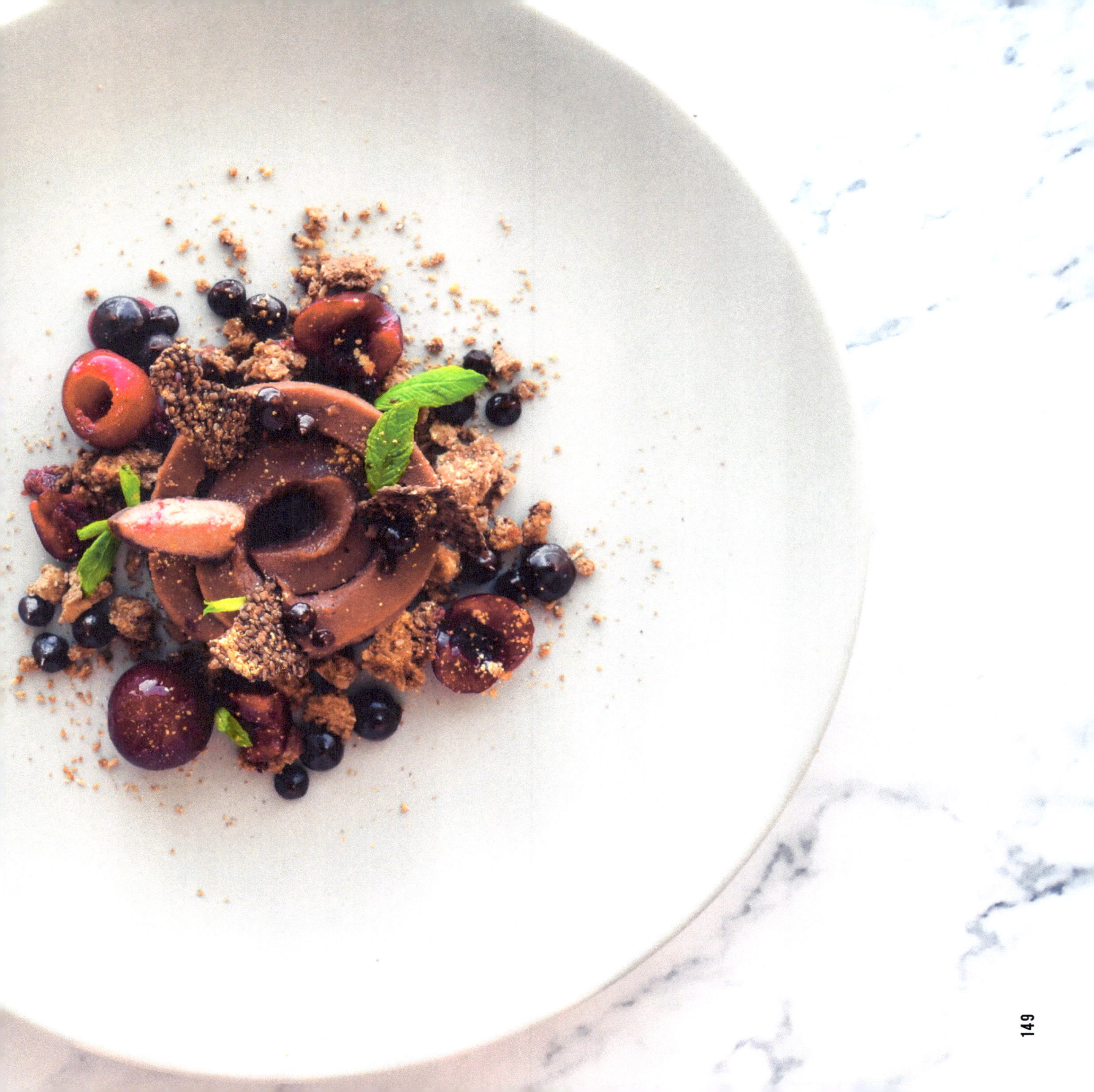

CHOCOLATE CHERRY SWIRL

Category - Pure-Raw + Dehydrated Raw
Time - 30 min prep + 12 hrs dehydration
Quantity - 2x15cm ring

Equipment - Food processor, dehydrator, 15cm and 6.5 cm ring cake moulds and piping bag

Chocolate Cherry Swirl

60 g cherry
30 g raw chocolate
1 tsp coconut oil
60 g coconut butter
60 g macadamia butter
50 ml coconut milk
40 g coconut sugar
1 tbsp lemon juice
A pinch of salt

To make custard

1. Blend the cherries in a high speed blender until puree, then transfer to your blender.
2. Melt the raw chocolate and coconut oil together over the water bath.
3. Add coconut butter, macadamia butter, coconut milk, coconut sugar, lemon juice and salt to your blender, blend with cherry puree.
4. Then add the melted raw chocolate and coconut oil. Blend again until well combined.
5. Pour mixture into 2x15 cm metal rings and set in the freezer for 1 hour.

Chocolate ganache
30 g raw chocolate
1 tbsp coconut milk

Decoration
Fresh cherries
Fresh mint
Edible gold powder

Other components
Graham soil - page 29
Chia tuile - page 173

Instructions for the chocolate ganache

1. Melt raw chocolate over the bain marie. Add coconut milk and mix well until smooth.
2. Transfer mixture into a small syringe. Set aside.

Assembly

1. Once chocolate cherry swirl cooled enough, pop the mousse from the rings. Transfer to a cold cutting board.
2. Using 6.5 cm metal ring cutter, cut out the centre of the mousse. You can use the centre later for a different recipe or eat to taste. We will not use the centre in this creation.
3. Now you have a 15cm round mousse; using a knife make it a longitudinal mousse by cutting off the edge of the ring. Then roll it. It will will be in the swirl shape as shown in the picture on page 149. Place onto a cold plate.
4. Crumble 3-4 tbsp graham soil around the swirl.
5. Make a circle by placing 4-5 cherries around the mousse.
6. Using a small syringe or piping bag, pipe the chocolate ganache in dots around the chocolate cherry swirl.
7. Using a chef tweezer, carefully place some small mint leaves between soil and cherries.
8. Break the chia tuile into 3 small pieces. Place it on top of the swirl leaving even space between them.
9. Pipe 2-3 small dots with chocolate ganache on the top of the swirl.
10. Dust some edible gold powder. Serve immediately!

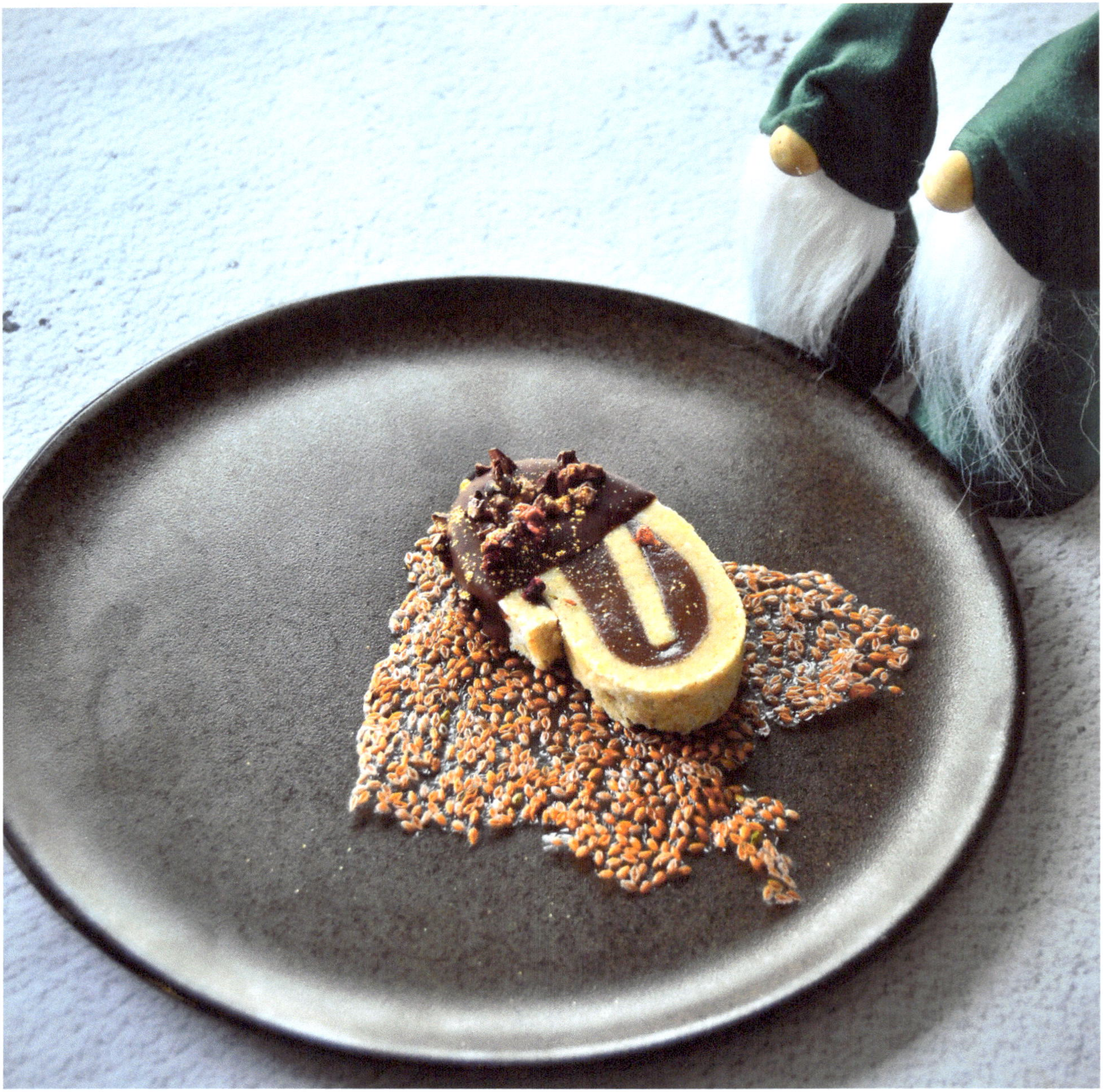

KOHLRABI NUTELLA SWISS ROLLS

Category - Dehydrated- Raw
Preperation - 40 min + 7 hrs dehydration
Quantity -5-7 person

Equipment - Blender, dehydrator
Personal note - Author's signature

Ingredients for the dough

200 g kohlrabi + 1/2 cup water
2 tbsp sesame oil
3 tbsp psyllium + 6 tbsp water
1 + 1/2 cup erythritol
1 cup water
40 g sprouted rolled oat flour
80 g almond flour
40 g coconut flour
1 tsp vanilla bean powder
1/2 tsp licorice salt

Instructions for the kohlrabi pastry dough

1. Place the sprouted rolled oats in the food processor, blend until you get powder.
2. Then add coconut flour, almond flour, licorice salt, vanilla powder and erythritol, combine together.
3. In a small bowl, mix psyllium husk powder with 6 tbsp water. Set aside for 5 minutes.
4. In a small food processor, make puree the kohlrabi with 1/2 cup water and sesame oil. Then transfer to food processor.
5. When psyllium gets sticky, transfer to your food processor.
6. Add the rest of the ingredients, blend until you get dough texture. Let it sit for 4-5 minutes until psyllium works well and everything is smooth.
7. Using 2 parchment papers and rolling pin, put the dough between papers and gently roll then cut it to size.
8. Dehydrate at 42° C for 6 -7 hours or until completely dried. After the first couple of hours you will need to flip it off the nonstick sheet so it dries directly on the mesh tray.

kohlrabi nutella swiss rolls continued

Ingredients for the nutella filling

1/2 cup unroasted hazelnut butter

1/4 cup coconut sugar

1/4 cup hazelnut milk

2 tbsp raw cacao powder

2 tbsp extra virgin olive oil

2 tbsp raw cacao butter, melted

1 tbsp coconut nectar syrup

1/2 tsp vanilla extract

A pinch of salt

Instructions

1. Place hazelnut butter into your Blendtec twister jar. Add the rest of the ingredients except cacao butter and olive oil. Blend well until well combined.
2. Lastly add the olive oil and cacao butter, blend again until smooth.
3. Let it sit in the refrigerator for 2 hours before using.

Ingredients for the psyllium tuile

1 tbsp psyllium seeds

4 tbsp water

Instructions

1. Place psyllium seeds in a small bowl, add the water. Mix and let it sit for 5-6 minutes.
2. Spread mixture over dehydrator sheets. Lay a very thin layer as much as possible.
3. Dehydrate until completely dried.

Ingredients for the chocolate sauce

100 g raw dark chocolate
2 tbsp raw cacao nibs

Assembly

1. Melt the raw chocolate using bain marie method. Set aside to cool a bit.
2. When the nutella has firmed up, spread the nutella over the dough. Dehydrate for 45-50 minutes.
3. Using a parchment paper, carefully roll the dough.
4. Place in the freezer for 2 hours before cutting it.
5. When it is cooled enough, cut and dip the half of swiss rolls in the melted chocolate. Spread raw cacao nibs and freeze dried raspberry pieces if desired. Store in the refrigerator in the airtight container up to couple of weeks.

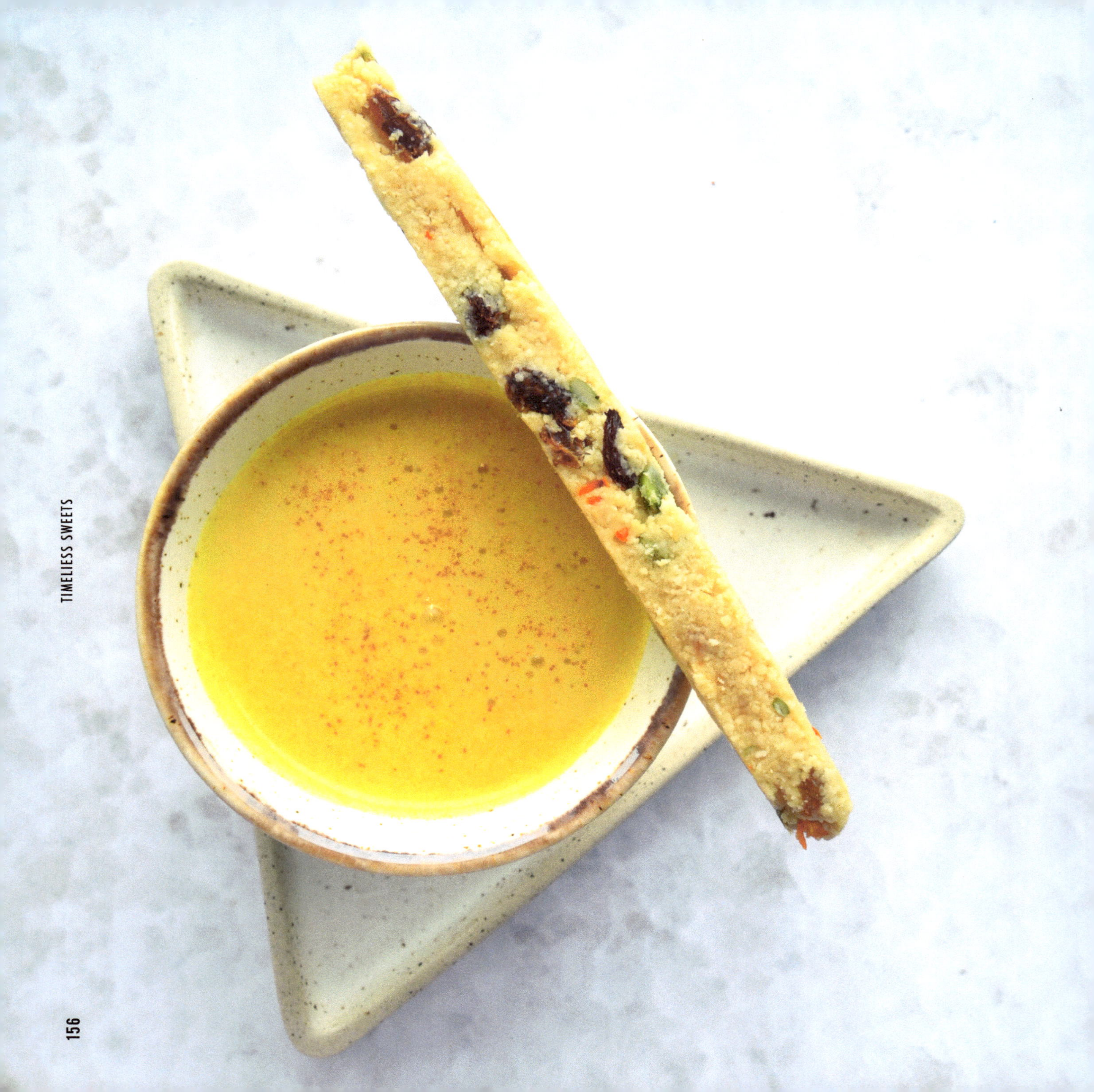

GOLDEN LATTE AND BISCOTTI

Category - Dehydrated- Raw
Preperation - 20 mins + 8 hrs dehydration
Equipment - Food processor, dehydrator, nut milk bag
Quantity - 2-3 person

Ingredients -Golden Latte

3 cups coconut milk
7 cm fresh turmeric
5 cm fresh ginger
1 tbsp maple syrup
1 tbsp almond butter
1/4 tsp pink himalayan salt

Biscotti

2 cups almond meal
1/4 cup maple syrup
1/2 cup dried raisins soaked
3 large medjool dates soaked
2 tbsp tahini
1/4 cup pumpkin seeds or pistachio
1/4 tsp pink himalayan salt

Instructions for the latte

1. Blend the warm coconut milk with the peeled turmeric and ginger and strain through a nut milk bag, vegan milker or sieve.
2. Add the sweetener, almond butter and a pinch of salt. Then blend again.
3. Sprinkle cinnamon and serve.

Notes:
If you don't have fresh turmeric and ginger, you can use 1/2 teaspoon of powder.

for the biscotti

1. Place all the ingredients in a large bowl. Mix by hand until throughly combined.
2. Divide the mixture in half and shape directly on dehydrator tray lined silicon paper into two long rectangles slightly mounded in the center.
3. Dehydrate at 46° C for 2 to 3 hours.
4. Once done, cut into bars about 2 cm wide.
5. Place bars to dehydrator, continue to dehydrate at 46° C for 6- 8 hours or until completely dried and slightly crispy.

SCANDINAVIAN FOREST CAKE

Category - Dehydrated-Raw
Time - 30 min prep + 16 hrs dehydration
Quantity - 15 cm ring cake

Equipment - Food processor, dehydrator

Kohlrabi crust ingredients

100 g kohlrabi
1 tbsp sesame oil
20 g oat flour
40 g almond flour
20 g coconut flour
1 tbsp psyllium powder
1/2 cup water
1 cup erythritol
1/2 cup cold brew rose hip tea

Cream ingredients

150 g raw cashews
4 tbsp lemon juice
3 tbsp maple syrup
1/2 cup coconut cream
1 tsp sunflower lecithin
1/4 tsp salt
2 tbsp cacao butter

Raspberry Jam

70 g frozen raspberries
30 g juniperberries
3/4 tsp psyllium powder

Other components

Graham soil (page 29)
Fresh strawberries or rasp-berries
Fresh mint

Chocolate layer

100 g raw chocolate
1/4 cup coconut milk
1 tbsp coconut oil
1 tbsp almond butter
1/4 tsp oak salt

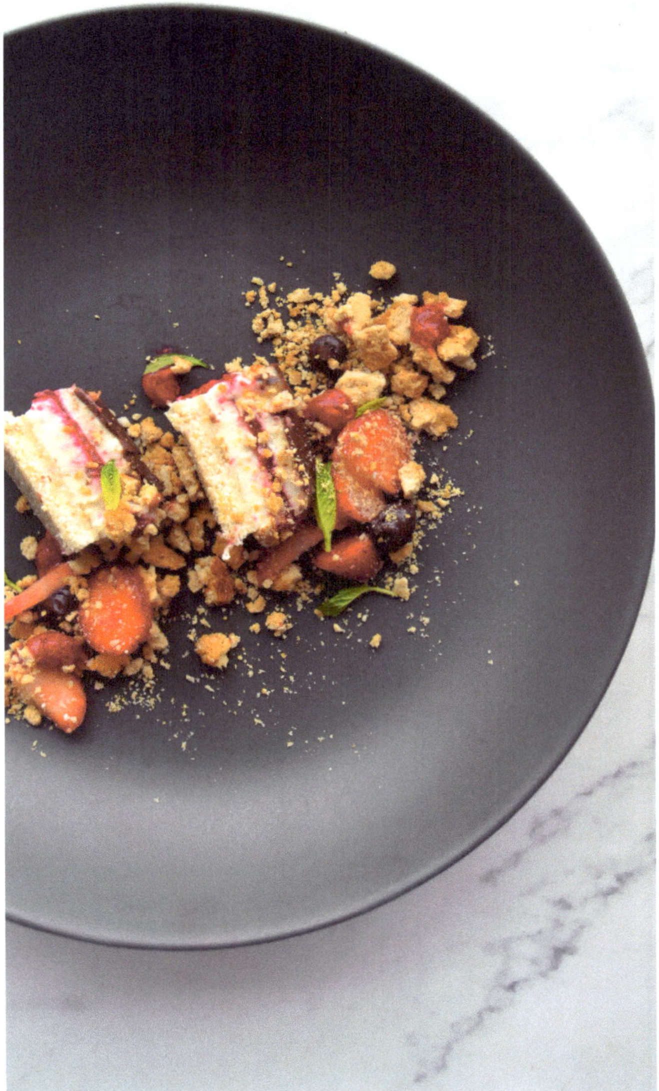

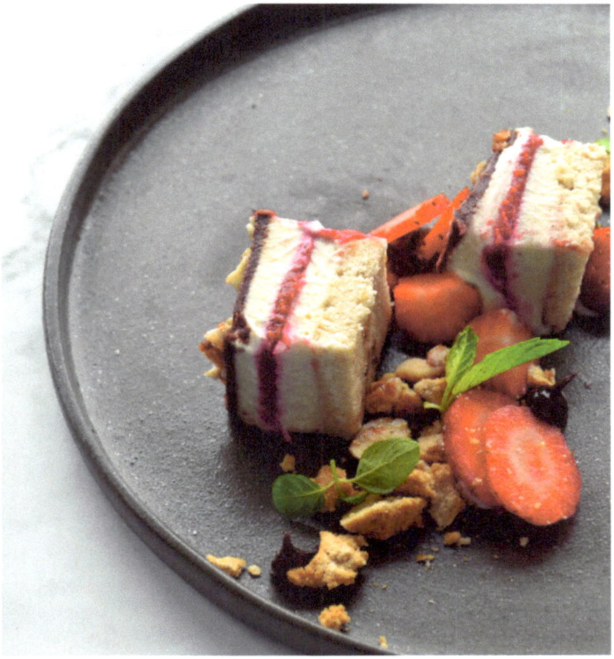

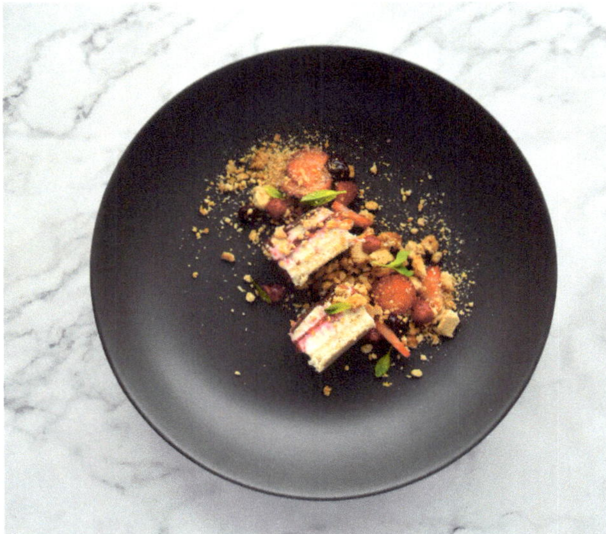

scandinavian forest cake continued

Instructions for the kohlrabi cake crust

1. Place the rolled oats in the food processor, blend well until you get powder.
2. Then add coconut flour, almond flour, licorice salt, vanilla powder and erythritol, combine together.
3. In a small bowl, mix psyllium husk powder with 6 tbsp water. Set aside for 5 minutes.
4. In a food processor, make puree the kohlrabi with 1/2 cup water and sesame oil.
5. When psyllium gets sticky, transfer to your food processor.
6. Add the rest of the ingredients, Blend until you get dough texture. Let it sit for 4-5 minutes until psyllium works well and everything is smooth.
7. Using 2 parchment paper and rolling pin, put the dough between papers and kindly roll and cut it to size.
8. Dehydrate at 42° C for 6 -7 hours or until completely dried. After the first couple of hours you will need to flip it off the nonstick sheet so it dries directly on the mesh tray.
9. Once done, using a 15cm ring cake mould, cut the dough in round shape, remove the edges; you can use keep them in the airtight container in the fridge to use later for different recipes.
10. Place the cake crust in a large bowl. Pour 1/2 cup rose-hip tea. Soak the crust for 1-2 minutes. Then immediately remove from the bowl and place onto a baking paper.

Instructions for the cream

1. Soak the cashews overnight or for 5-6 hours. Then strain and and transfer to a high speed blender.
2. Add the lemon juice, coconut cream, lecithin, salt and maple. Blend well until silky smooth.
3. Melt the raw cacao butter over a water bath using a thermometer to keep it around maximum 42° C.
4. Once melted, pour into your mixture. Blend again until well combined.

Instructions for the raspberry jam

1. Place raspberries and juniperberries into your blender. Blend until puree. Transfer to a small bowl.
2. Add the psyllium powder and using a spoon, mix well.
3. Let it sit for 20-30 minutes or until thick.

Instructions for the chocolate sauce

1. Melt raw chocolate over the water bath.
2. Add the rest of ingredients and blend until thick.

Assembly

1. Place 15cm cake mould on the crust.
2. Pour the half of the cream over the crust.
3. Place to your freezer for 1 hour.
4. Once gets cold, pour the raspberry jam over the cream. Spread well.
5. Keep in the freezer for 30 minutes.
6. Then pour the remaining half of the cream over the jam.
7. Now set in the freezer for 2 hours.
8. Remove cake from the mould.
9. Lay a baking paper on your surface.
10. Place a baking tray, then place cake over the tray.
11. Set aside 1-2 tbsp chocolate to use it for the plating later. Then pour the chocolate sauce over the cake, make sure it is coated well.
12. Let it cool for 15-20 minutes then transfer to a small plate and set in the freezer for 2 hours.
13. After 2 hours, remove cake from the freezer, using a sharp and hot knife, slice it into squares or how you prefer.
14. Place 2 square in a plate. Add the almond soil, fresh strawberries or raspberries and mint. Using a pipping bag, squeeze small chocolate dots around the cake. Serve immediately.

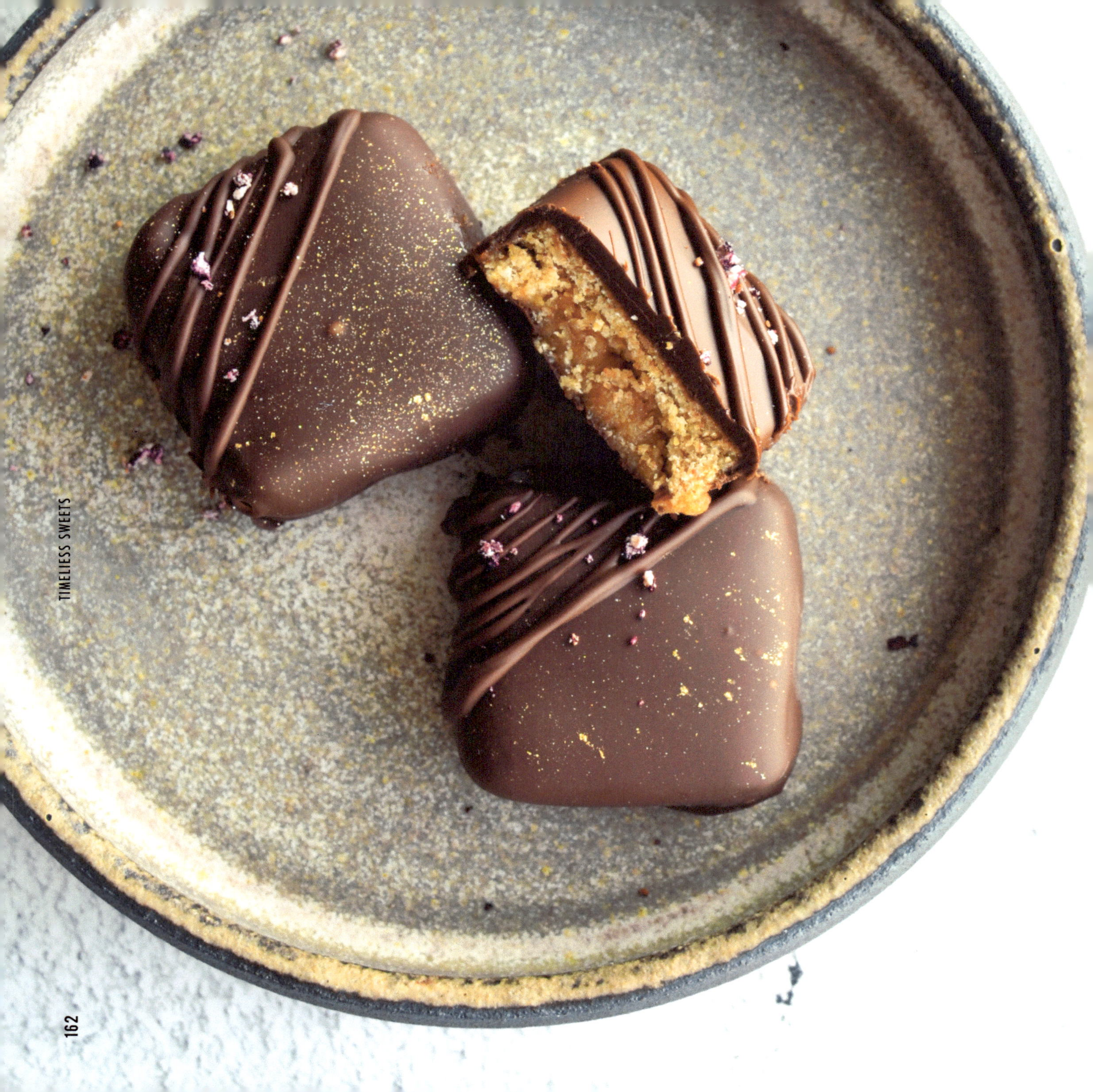

OAT CARAMEL BISCUITS

Category - Pure-Raw
Time - 30 min prep
Quantity - 15 biscuits

Equipment - Blender, dehydrator, 3cm square cutter
Personal note - A perfect blend of salty and sweet and a little bite of heaven!

Oat cookie base

1 cup oats blended into flour
1/2 cup buckini blended into flour
1/2 tsp baking powder
1/4 tsp salt
4 tbsp desiccated coconut
2 tbsp coconut sugar
80 g maple syrup
2 tsp vanilla bean powder
2 tbsp water

Coconut caramel

100 g medjool dates, measured after seeds removed
55 g almond butter
1 tsp vanilla bean powder
65 g coconut cream
1 tbsp maple syrup
1/4 tsp salt

Chocolate shell

50 g raw cacao butter
4 tbsp coconut oil
1/2 cup raw cacao powder
2 tbsp maple syrup
A pinch salt

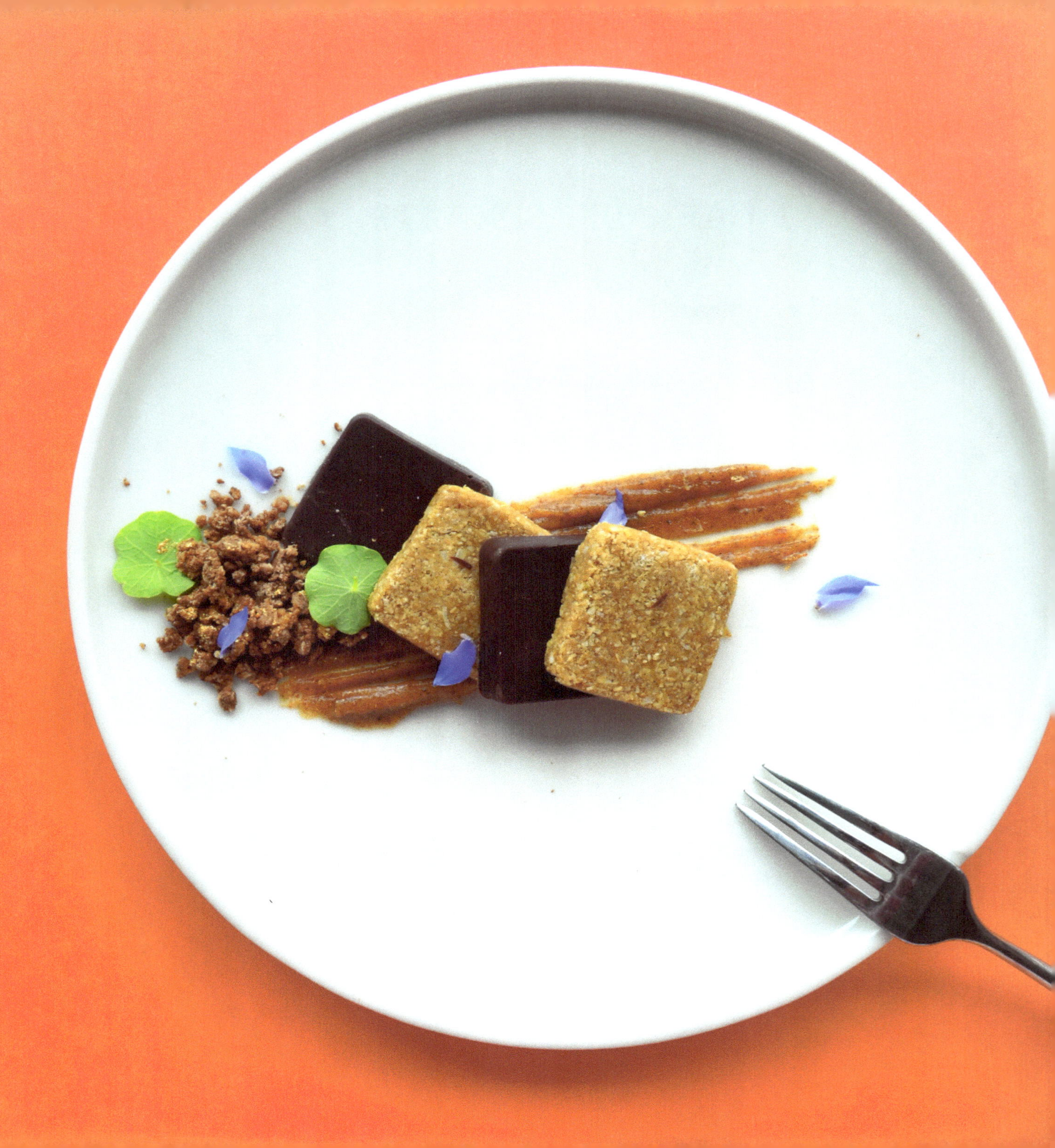

To make cookie base

1. Simply whisk together the dry ingredients (oats, baking powder, salt and coconut) before stirring through the maple syrup and vanilla.
2. Roll out between two sheets of baking paper to about the thickness of the metal tip of a pen (3-5mm).
3. Cut out with a 3cm square cookie cutter before transferring to a lined baking tray. Bake at dehydrator at 42° C for 4-5 hours and then transfer to your working space while you prepare the other elements.

To make caramel

1. To make caramel, drain the water off the dates before adding them to a blender with the remaining ingredients.
2. Blend on high speed until super smooth, scraping down the sides as necessary. Set aside.

To make chocolate shell

1. Place cacao butter and coconut oil over a double boiler. Set aside to melt completely, stirring occasionally.
2. Once melted, whisk through the cacao powder, followed by the maple syrup and salt. Leave the chocolate over the double-boiler at 42° C while you're assembling the cookies, as this will make it easier to work with.

Assembly

1. Top each oat biscuit with a heaped tablespoon of caramel, spreading evenly to the edges with a knife. Place on a plate and freeze for at least 30 minutes (this will make them easier to coat in the chocolate).
2. Lower each caramel-topped biscuit into the chocolate with a fork, allowing the excess to drip back into the bowl.
3. Place each coated biscuit back on the plate and allow to set in the fridge for 10-15 minutes.

Tip: To make this dessert deconstructed; pour date caramel on the plate, lay the chocolate and cookie base. Add almond soil, garnish with nasturtium and borage. See the picture on the left page.

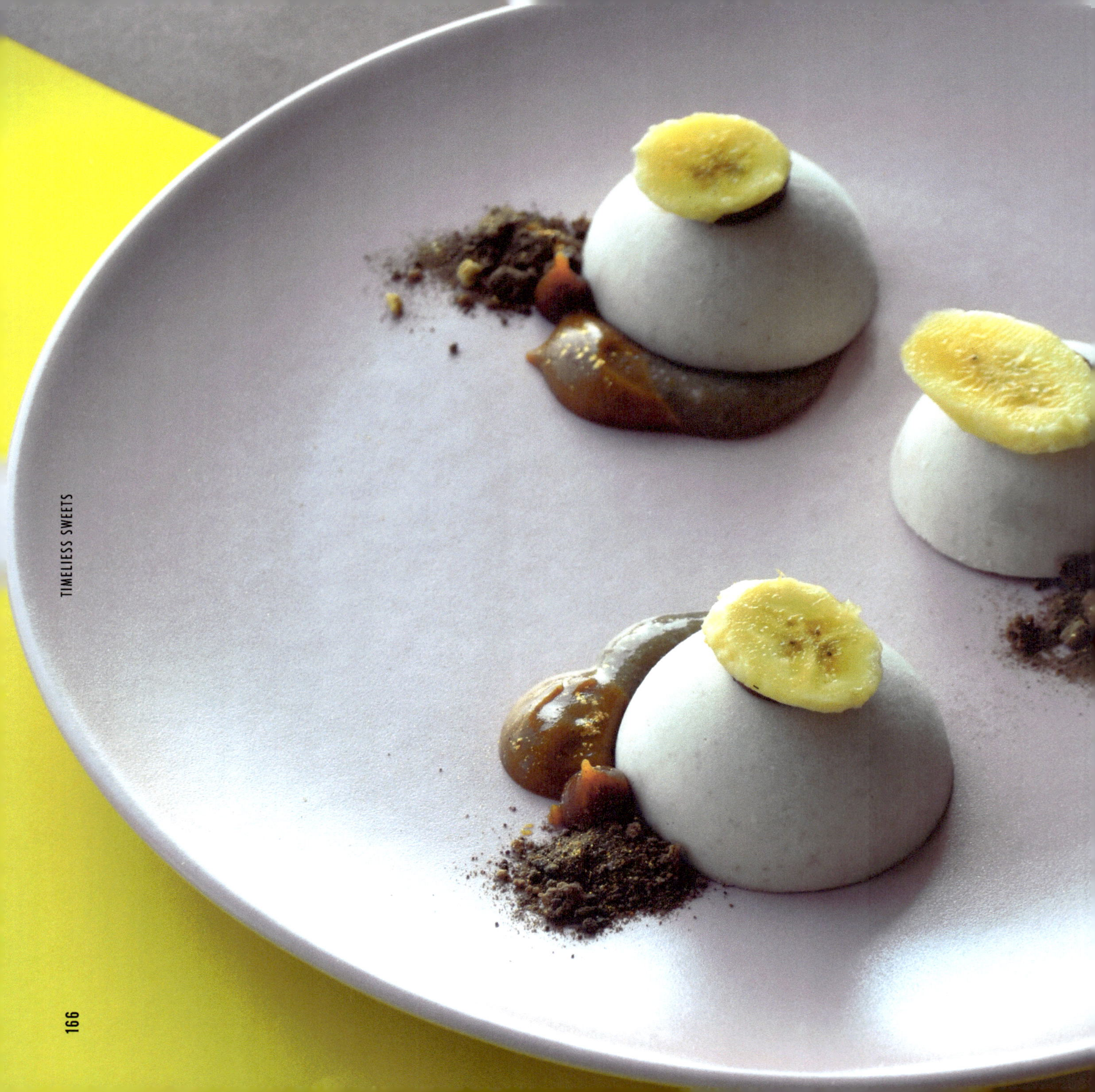

DECONSTRUCTED BANOFFEE

Category - Pure-Raw + Dehydrated Raw
Time - 1 hour prep + 8 hrs dehydration
Quantity - 3-4 plates

Equipment - Blender, non-stick sheets, spatula, dehydrator, 5cm ring molds
Personal note - Brings childhood memories

Salted Tahini Caramel

5 medjool dates (70g measured after seeds removed)
40 ml water
1 tbsp lime juice
2 tbsp coconut sugar
1 tbsp tahini
1 tbsp coconut butter
1/4 tsp licorice salt
1/4 tsp cinnamon powder

Toffee Soil

1/2 cup almond butter (80g)
2 tbsp cacao butter
1 tbsp carob powder
2 tbsp brazil nut milk
2 tbsp coconut sugar
1 tbsp lucuma

Banana Caramel

2 tbsp coconut butter
3 semi-frozen bananas
1 tbsp lucuma
1/4 tsp licorice salt

Banana Pecan Cheesecake

120g pecan nuts soaked
1/4 cup pecan milk
1 tbsp lime juice
2 tbsp maple syrup
2 drops medicine flower banana extract
2 tbsp cacao butter melted
A pinch salt

Decoration

Sliced fresh bananas
Edible gold powder (optional)
Borage (optional)

deconstructed banoffee continued

To make the tahini salted caramel

1. Soak dates in warm water for 10-15 minutes, then strain, dry and transfer to your blender.
2. Add the water, lime juice, coconut sugar, tahini, salt & coconut butter.
3. Blend until silky smooth. It should be a slightly thick pourable mixture.

To make toffee soil

1. Place all the toffee soil ingredients into your blender, blend until smooth. Set the 1/4 of the mixture to pipe later.
2. Pour the rest onto the dehydrator tray lined silicon paper. Dehydrate at 42° C for 12-14 hours or until completely dried.
3. Once done, place shards to a small food processor. Blend to get soil. You may want to leave chunky pieces. Do not blend too much.

To make the banana pecan caramel

1. Place semi-frozen bananas into a high speed blender. Add the coconut butter, lucuma and licorice salt.
2. Blend until you get a slightly thick liquid mixture. (If the mixture is too runny, you may need to add a bit psyllium husk powder to make it thicker.)

To make the banana cheesecake

1. Place all the banana pecan caramel ingredients except cacao butter in the blender. Blend until silky smooth. Then add the melted cacao butter blend again until well combined.
2. Pour mixture into the 5cm ring moulds. Freeze for 2-3 hours.

Assembly

1. Pour 3 tablespoons of caramel into the plate, leaving a space between them to create a ring.
2. Pour 3 tablespoons of banana caramel next to the tahini caramel.
3. Remove cheesecake moulds from the freezer. Place 3 banana cheesecake pieces onto the caramel rings.
4. Pipe a dot from the tahini salted caramel on the cheesecake pieces.
5. Place sliced banana pieces onto the banana cheesecakes.
6. Gently sprinkle the soil next to the caramel. Serve immediately!

SWISS CHOCOLATE MOUSSE

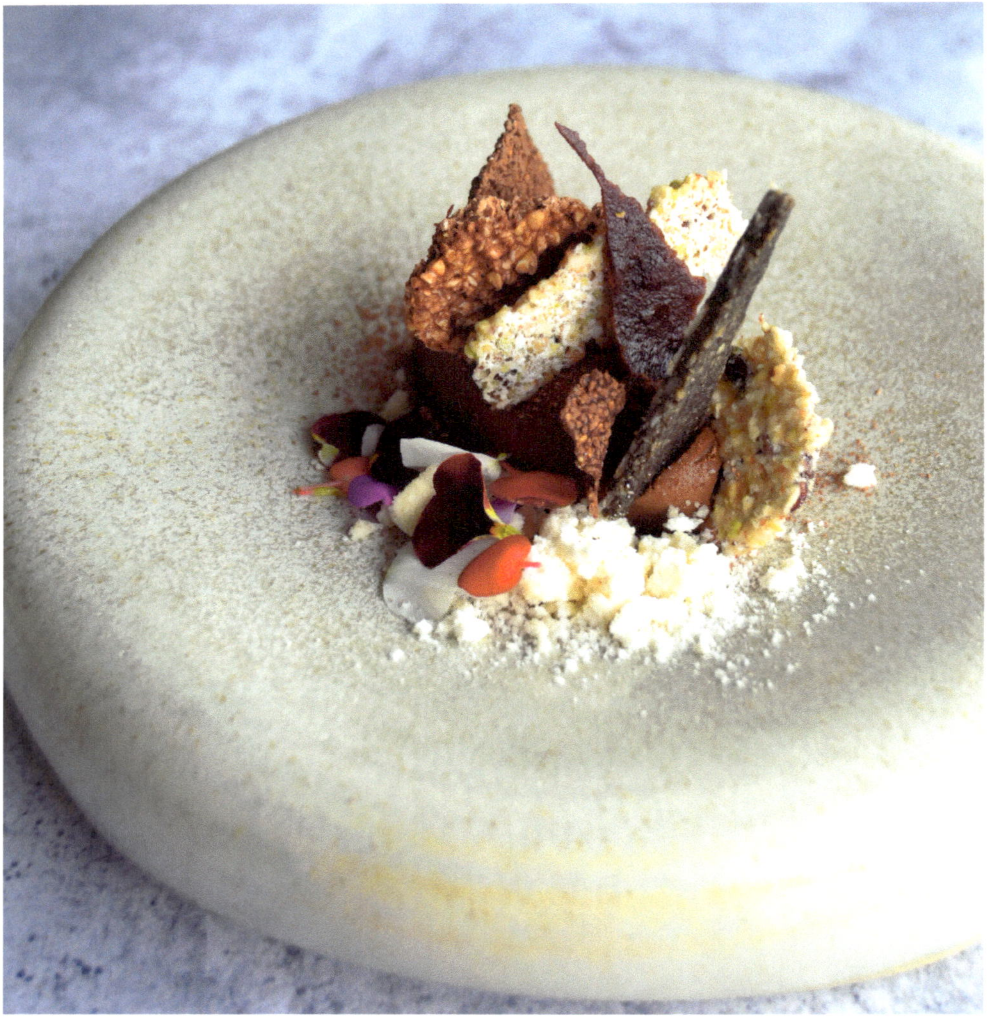

with 4 texture crisps

Four different dehydrated 'crisps' created using chia seeds, dates and, dried raisins and nuts. This is an easy but impressive looking dessert that's perfect for any season.

Category - Pure Raw
Preperation - 20 minutes
Makes - 6-8 quenelle mousse

Equipment - Blender, dehydrator, and quenelle moulds

Mousse ingredients

250 g hass type avocados
160 g raw dark chocolate
100 ml homemade almond milk
1 tbsp raw cacao powder
A pinch of pink himalayan salt

Instructions

1. Peel your avocados, remove the seed.
2. Place soaked avocados, cacao powder and pinch of salt into a high speed blender. Blend until smooth.
3. Place the raw dark chocolate and coconut oil into a small bowl. Place this bowl in to a larger bowl of hot water and melt together with the occasional stir. If you wish for the recipe to remain 'completely raw', monitor the heat with a thermometer to maintain under 42° C.
4. Once melted add the chocolate mix to ingredients already in the blender. Blend until fully incorporated.
5. Pour into quenelle moulds and set in fridge overnight. For crisps, continue with the next pages.

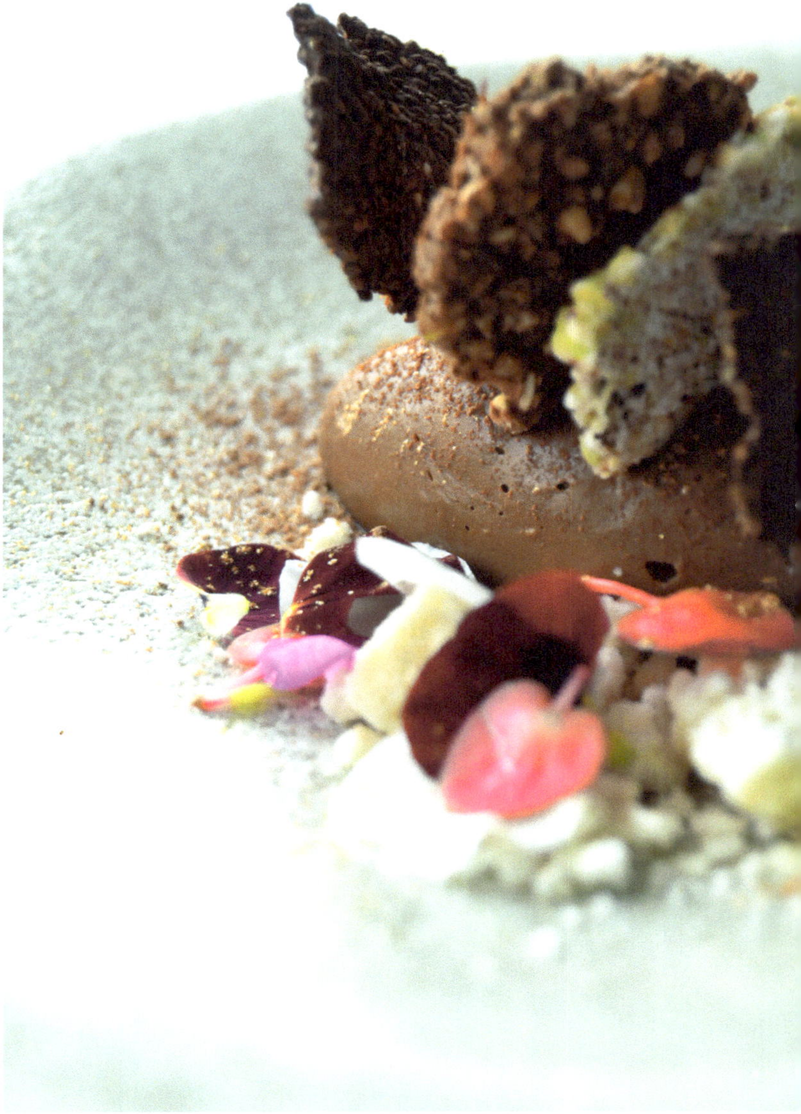

DATE CRISP

Category - Dehydrator

Dehydration - approx. 8-10 hours

Equipment - blender, spatula, dehydrator

Makes - 30x30 1 dehydrator sheet

Ingredients

80 g medjool dates

65 g water

1 tbsp raw cacao powder

A pinch of pink himalayan salt

Instructions

1. Soak your dates in the water for 30 minutes. Then strain the water.
2. Place the dates and all the ingredients into a high speed blender and blend until smooth.
3. Spread mixture nice and thinly on to a dehydrator tray lined with a silicon mat and dehydrate at 43° C overnight or for 8-10 hours in the dehydrator.
4. Flip on to mesh tray and dehydrate for another couple of hours.
5. Peel off tray and allow to cool. Once cooled, break into shards.

CHIA CRISP

Category - Dehydrator
Dehydration - approx. 6-8 hours
Equipment - blender, spatula, dehydrator
Makes - 30x30 1 dehydrator sheet

Ingredients

35 g chia seeds
2 tbsp coconut sugar
150 g coconut milk or water
2 tbsp raw cacao powder

Instructions

1. Place all ingredients into a bowl and stir to combine.
2. Allow to sit for 2 hours, until mixture is thick and the chia has absorbed most of the liquid.
3. Spread mixture on to a dehydrator tray lined with a silicon mat and dehydrate at 42° C overnight or for 6-8 hours in a dehydrator.
4. Allow to cool.
5. Once cooled, break into shards.

VANILLA BUCKWHEAT CRISP

Category - Dehydrator
Dehydration - approx. 8-10 hours
Makes - 30x30 1 dehydrator sheet

Equipment - food processor, spatula, dehydrator
Storage - in an airtight container up to 2-3 weeks.

Ingredients

1 cup buckwheat soaked
50 g maple syrup
1 tsp vanilla powder
1/4 tsp salt

Instructions

1. Soak raw buckwheats in the water for 1 hour, then strain and drain. Transfer to your food processor.
2. Add the maple syrup, vanilla and salt.
3. Process until well combined but not throughly pureed.
4. Divide mixture between silicon lined dehydrator trays and spread to about 3mm thickness.
5. Dehydrate at 46° C for 6-7 hours or until completely dried.
6. You may need to flip it and continue to dehydrate additional 1-2 hours until completely crispy.
7. Once done, break into pieces. They are ready to eat.

swiss chocolate mousse continued

Add-on crisp ideas

- Oat meal thins recipe also can be served with this mousse.
- Add the cacao or carob powder to the vanilla buckwheat crisp recipe to make it chocolatey.

Assembly

1. To serve, remove chocolate mousse from the quenelle moulds. Place in a white handmade stoneware plate.
2. Break up the crisps and serve each one on the top of your mousse. They can be used as your spoon.

OAT HAZELNUT CRISP

Category - Dehydrator
Dehydration - approx. 8-10 hours
Makes - 30x30 1 dehydrator sheet

Equipment - food processor, spatula, dehydrator
Storage - in an airtight container up to 1-2 months.

Ingredients

80 g gluten-free sprouted rolled oats
10 g chia seeds
135 g hazelnut butter
1-2 tbsp plant milk (or water)
3 tbsp maple
A pinch salt

Instructions

1.Place the oats, chia seeds and salt in the food processor, blitz until slightly flour.
2. Add the hazelnut butter, maple and plant milk. Process until everything combined well. You should get a sticky dough.
3. Using two parchment paper and a rolling pin, roll the dough between parchment, as thin as possible. Transfer to a dehydrator tray.
4. Dehydrate ifor 8-10 hours. Then flip and continue to dehydrate until completely dried and crispy. Enjoy alone or serve your raw cakes.

FERRAWRO NO SHARE

Category - Dehydrated-Raw
Dehydration time - 12 hours

Equipment - Food processor, dehydrator, 2.5 cm half-sphere mould
Serves - 15 pieces

Wafer

1/4 cup walnut flour
1/4 cup almond flour
2 tbsp coconut butter
1/4 cup oat flour
70 g medjool dates

Gianduja ganache

1/2 cup hazelnut butter
5 tbsp coconut sugar
2 tbsp raw cacao powder
2 tbsp raw cacao butter
1/8 tsp vanilla bean powder
2 tbsp coconut milk
A pinch salt

Chocolate coating

70 g raw dark chocolate
1 tsp coconut oil
1/2 cup chopped hazelnuts

Hazelnut core

15 hazelnuts

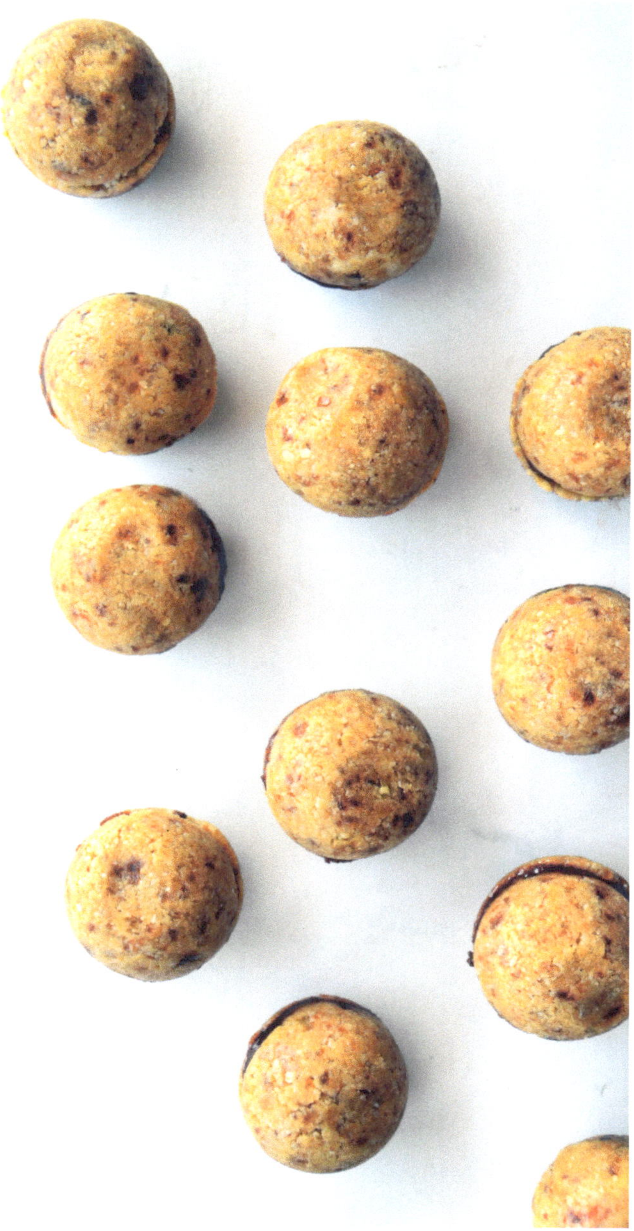

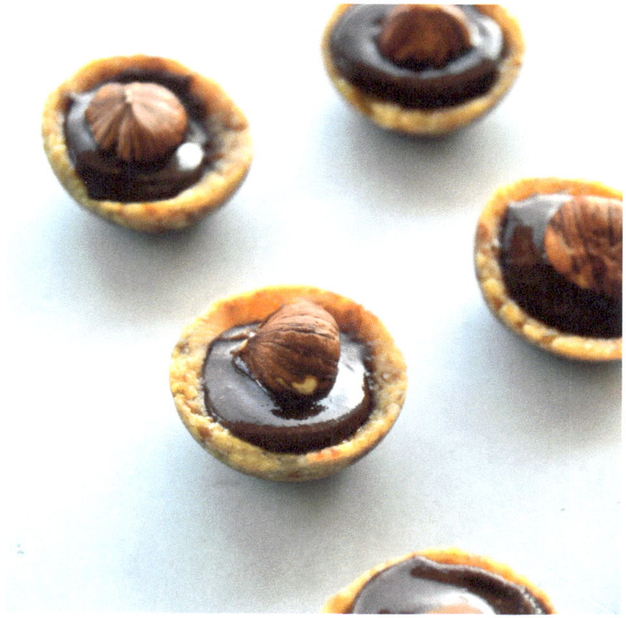

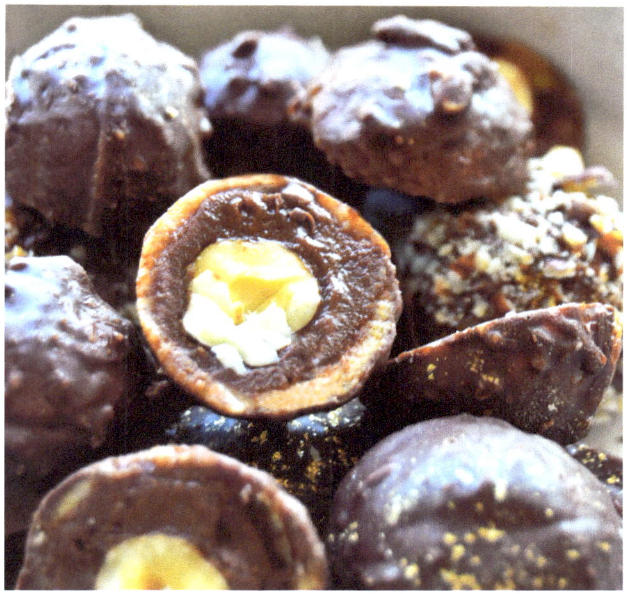

ferrawro no share continued

To make wafer

1. Add all the ingredients into food processor. Blend until you get dough form.
2. Press the dough into a half-sphere mould about 4 g per hole.
3. Place the mold in the dehydrator and dehydrate at 42°C for 4-5 hours, then carefully remove the mold and place dough pieces on the dehydrator tray lined silicon paper.
4. Continue to dehydrate for 10-12 hours or until completely crispy.

To make gianduja

1. In a blender, combine the hazelnut butter and coconut sugar. Blend to a smooth butter consistency.
2. Then add the cacao powder, melted cacao butter, vanilla and salt. Blend until well combined. Add the warm water. Blend again until well combined.
3. Transfer the mixture into a bowl. Fill the shells until almost full, leaving some allowance for the hazelnut core.
4. Return the mold to the freezer to set partially, about 15-20 minutes, so that the ganache is still soft enough to press in a hazelnut.

Assembly

1. Press a hazelnut into half of the spheres 30 pieces in total , and make an indentation in the remaining half.
2. Return the mold to the freezer and allow to set fully.
3. Unmold the shells and join a half with the hazelnut to another half with an indentation. You should have about 15 full spheres now.
4. Melt the raw chocolate over bain marie. Add the coconut oil and mix well. Stir in chopped hazelnuts.
5. Using a chocolate fork, gently dip each sphere into the chocolate. Place on a parchment paper and immediately sprinkle more crushed hazelnuts over. Repeat with the rest of the balls.
6. Keep in the refrigerator for 1 hour before serving.

WALNUT PANNA COTTA WITH MULLED STRAWBERRIES

Category - Pure-Raw +Dehydrated-Raw
Time - 30 min prep + 12 hrs dehydration

Equipment - Blender, dehydrator, 4.5 or 5cm half sphere moulds
Quantity - 2-3 person

Panna cotta ingredients

100 g walnuts
70 g coconut cream
3 tbsp maple syrup
50 ml coconut milk
30 g coconut oil
1 tbsp lemon juice
1 tbsp rose water
A pinch salt

Mulled strawberries

1 cup fresh strawberries
1 kiwi cubed
5 cm fresh ginger cubed
1 tsp vanilla bean powder
1 tsp maple syrup
A few peels of lemon and orange zest
Juice of 1 lemon
Fresh basil leaves
Edible gold powder to dust

Black sesame brittle

1 cup black sesame seeds
1/4 cup coconut sugar
1/4 cup maple syrup
A pinch salt
OR
use coconut lace tuile (recipe on the page 184)

walnut panna cotta with mulled strawberries continued

To make the panna cotta

1. To make the panna cotta, place all ingredients, excluding the coconut oil in a blender and blend until very smooth.
2. Slowly add coconut oil with the blender still running and continue blending until it emulsifies into the mixture.
3. Divide panna cotta mixture between 2-3 glasses and leave in the fridge to set for 4-5 hours.

To make the mulled strawberries

1. For the mulled strawberries, slice the strawberries into quarters and place in a bowl along with the rest of the ingredients.
2. Leave in the fridge for 2-4 hours to mull.

To make the black sesame brittle

1. Using a coffee grinder, grind the coconut sugar. Transfer to a bowl.
2. Add the black sesame seeds and maple. Give it a good toss.
3. Spread mixture onto the dehydrator tray lined silicon sheet.
4. Dehydrate at 42° C until completely dried and crispy.

Alternatively you can use coconut lace tuile on the page 184. They both taste good with the panna cotta.

Assembly

To serve, remove lemon zest from the strawberries. Using a strainer, strain them. Take one quarter of the strawberry mixture and blend until smooth, then fold back through the rest of the mulled strawberries. Divide between the set panna cottas, add the cubed kiwis, ginger and the rest of the strawberries. Decorate with peeled lemon and orange zest and fresh basil leaves.

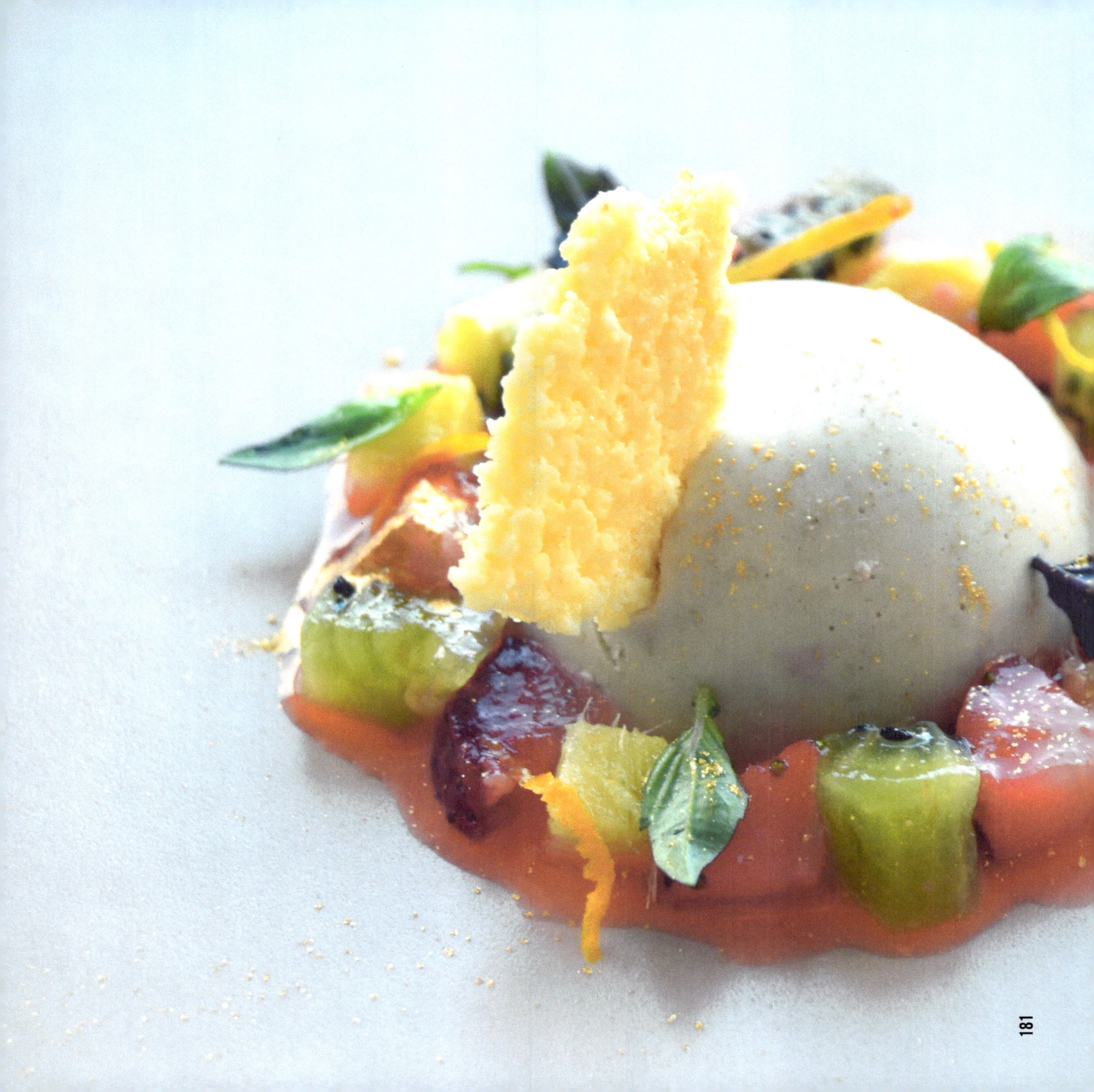

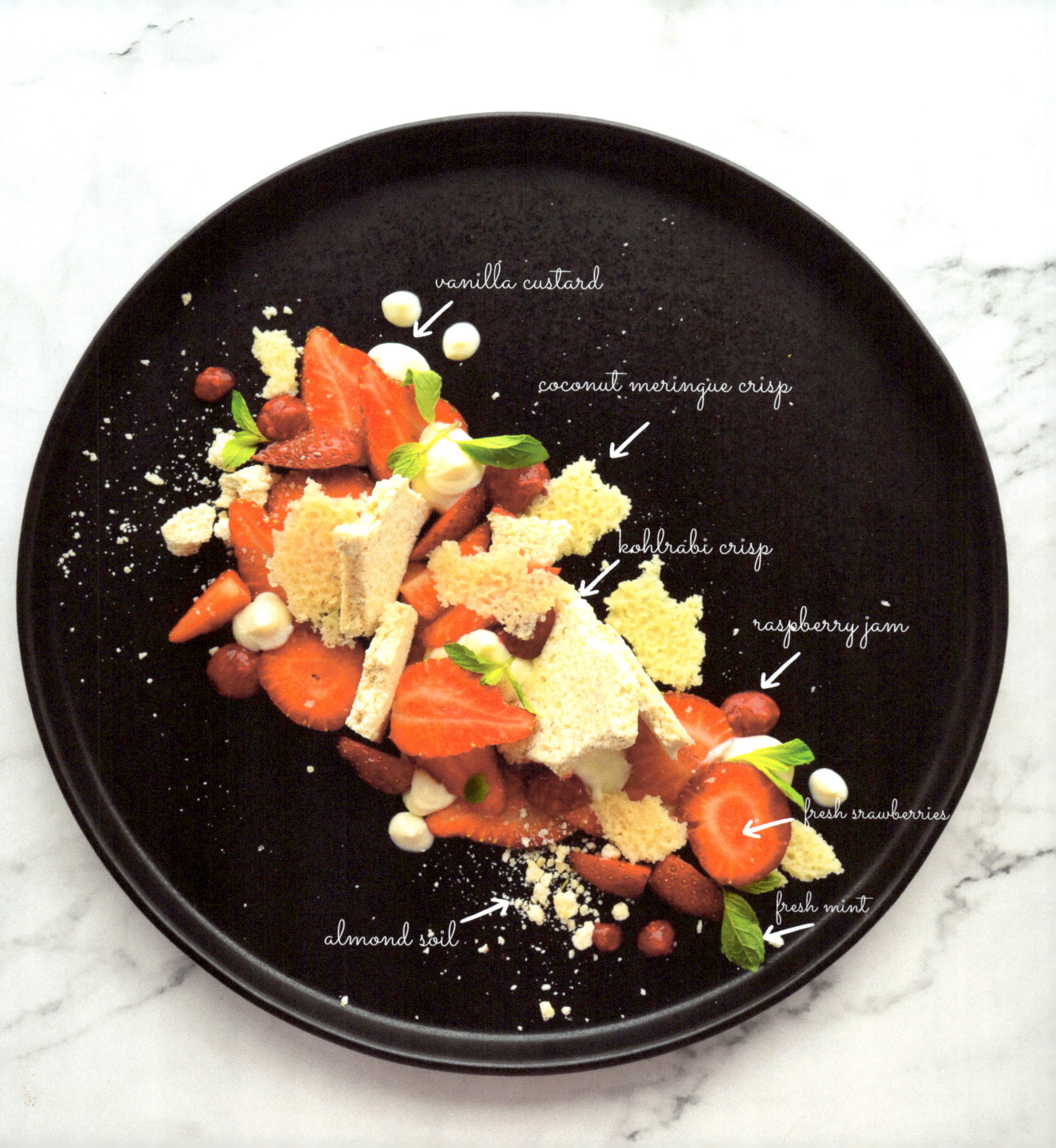
vanilla custard
coconut meringue crisp
kohlrabi crisp
raspberry jam
fresh srawberries
fresh mint
almond soil

DECONSTRUCTED PAVLOVA

Category - Dehydrated-Raw
Time - 20 min prep + 28 hrs dehydration
Quantity - 2-3 plates

Equipment - Food processor, blender,dehydrator
Personal note - A wonderful sensory experience

Vanilla custard ingredients
100 g young coconut meat
1/4 cup coconut water
1 tsp vanilla bean powder
3 tbsp lemon juice
1 tbsp coconut oil

Raspberry jam ingredients
50 g fresh raspberries
1/2 tsp psyllium powder

Other components
Coconut meringue crisp (page 184)
Kohlrabi crisp (use kohlrabi crust recipe on the page 163, just dehydrate longer)
White almond soil (page 29)
Fresh mint and strawberries

To make custard
1. Place all custard ingredients except coconut oil into your blender. Blend until silky smooth. Then add the coconut oil, blend until well combined.
2. Pour mixture in a pipping bag. We will use to pipe the custard around the kohlrabi and meringue crisps.

To make raspberry jam
1. Place raspberries into a blender, blend until puree.
2. Then add the psyllium and let it sit for 20 minutes until psyllium absorbs the water and the mixture is thick enough to pipe. Once done. Transfer to a pipping bag.

Assembly
1. Slice fresh strawberries thinly, place on a large plate randomly.
2. Pipe the vanilla custard.
3. Cut the kohlrabi crisps and coconut meringue crisps randomly, add on your plate.
4. Pipe some raspberry jam dots between the crisps.
5. Sprinkle white almond soil. Decorate with fresh mint.

deconstructed pavlova continued

COCONUT MERINGUE CRISP (LACE TUILE)

Category - Dehydrated-Raw
Time - 8 min prep + 24 hrs dehydration
Quantity - 15cm dehydrator tray

Equipment - blender, non-stick sheets, spatula, dehydrator
Personal note - heavenly versatile crisp!

Ingredients

100 g coconut cream
2 tbsp coconut nectar or maple syrup
1/2 cup desiccated coconut
1/2 tsp vanilla extract

Instructions

1. Refrigerate your coconut cream overnight.
2. In the morning scoop the solid cream off the top, discarding the water left in the can.
3. Place solid cream into your blender. Add all the remaining ingredients. Blend well until well combined.
4. Pour the mixture onto dehydrator tray lined silicon sheets.
5. Dehydrate for 19-20 hrs until dried and easily turnable, remove the silicon sheet and continue to dehydrate back side for about 4-6 hours or until fully dried and crispy.
6. Once crispy, break into shards. Keep in the refrigerator. Once refrigerated for 2 hours, they become harder and crispier as we want, then they are ready to decorate!

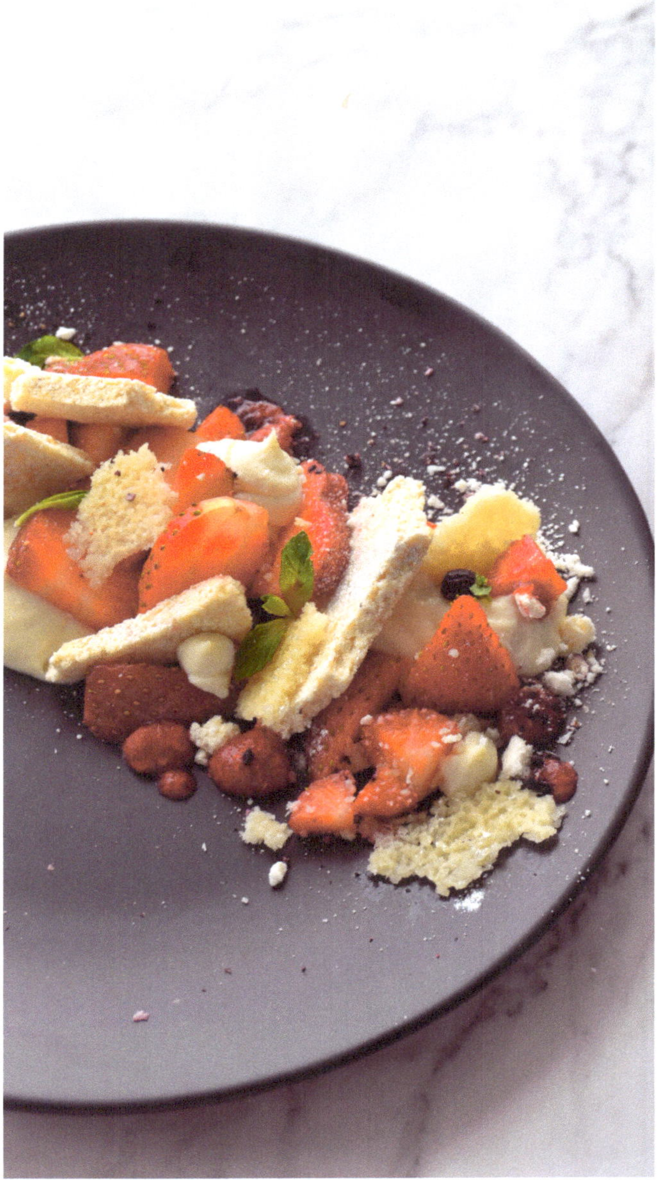

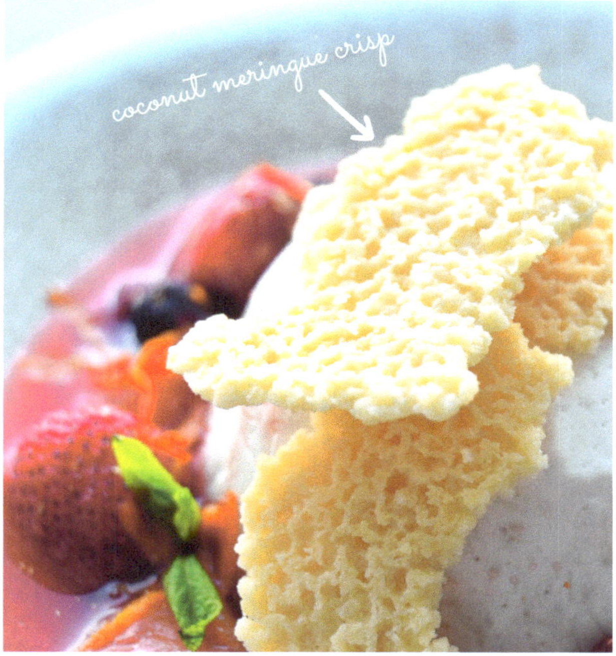
coconut meringue crisp

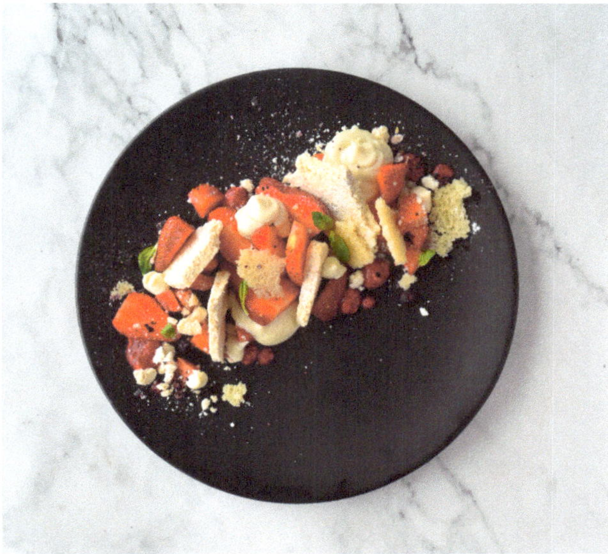

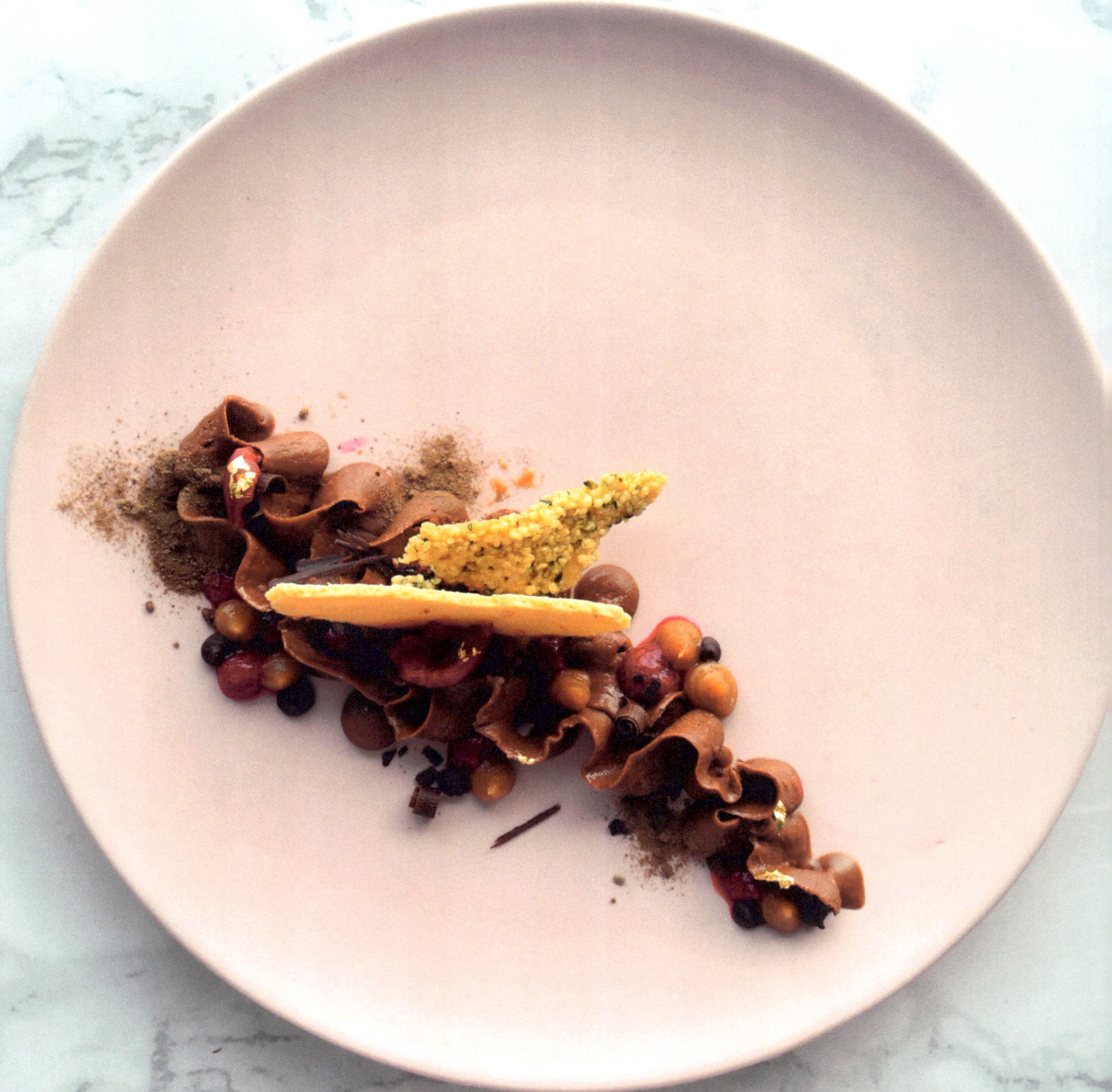

GIANDUIOTTO RIBBON

Category - Pure-Raw + Dehydrated Raw
Time - 1 hour prep + 8 hrs dehydration
Quantity - 3-4 plates

Equipment - Blender, non-stick sheets, spatula, dehydrator, Ateco 150 ribbon pastry tube, pipping bag
Deconstructed form of Italian classic

Gianduiotto ribbon
75 g raw chocolate
150 g hazelnut butter

Cherry Fluid Gel
1 cup cherries
1 tbsp agave or maple
1 tsp psyllium husk powder

Black chocolate soil
1 tbsp coconut sugar
1 tbsp raw cacao nibs
1/8 tsp charcoal powder

Other components
Fresh cherries halved
Shaved raw dark chocolate
Edible gold leaf

Hemp snap
1/2 cup hemp hearts
2 tbsp light agave or maple syrup

Salted Caramel
1 cup medjool dates soaked
2 tbsp nut butter of choice
2 tbsp plant milk
1/4 tsp licorice salt (from Saltverk Iceland) or miso

Meringue Shard
70 g macadamia soaked
2 tbsp lemon juice
1 tbsp light agave or coconut nectar
1 tbsp cacao butter
A pinch salt

gianduiotto ribbon continued

On the previous page, for the gianduiotto you use store-bought raw hazelnut butter and raw chocolate, as well as you can make them yourself from scratch. If you are going to make from scratch, check this page. Otherwise, you can go to the next page.

Hazelnut butter from scratch

150 g raw hazelnut

Raw chocolate from scratch

90 g raw cacao butter
60 g raw cacao paste
1/2 tsp vanilla powder
25 g coconut sugar powdered

To make the hazelnut butter

1. To make raw hazelnut butter, soak hazelnuts overnight. In the morning, strain and drain them. Place in the dehydrator. Heat at 42° C until they are completely dried.
2. Place nuts in the Blendtec twister jar. Process on high speed until completely smooth and you get batter scraping down the sides as needed. It may take 2-3 minutes.

To make the chocolate

1. Melt cocoa paste and cacao butter in a large bowl using the bain marie method over medium-low heat.
2. When the temperature reaches 37° C, add coconut nectar syrup, salt and vanilla and continue whisking.
3. Spread the mixture evenly as thin as possible on a parchment paper.
4. Store in the refrigerator until ready to serve.

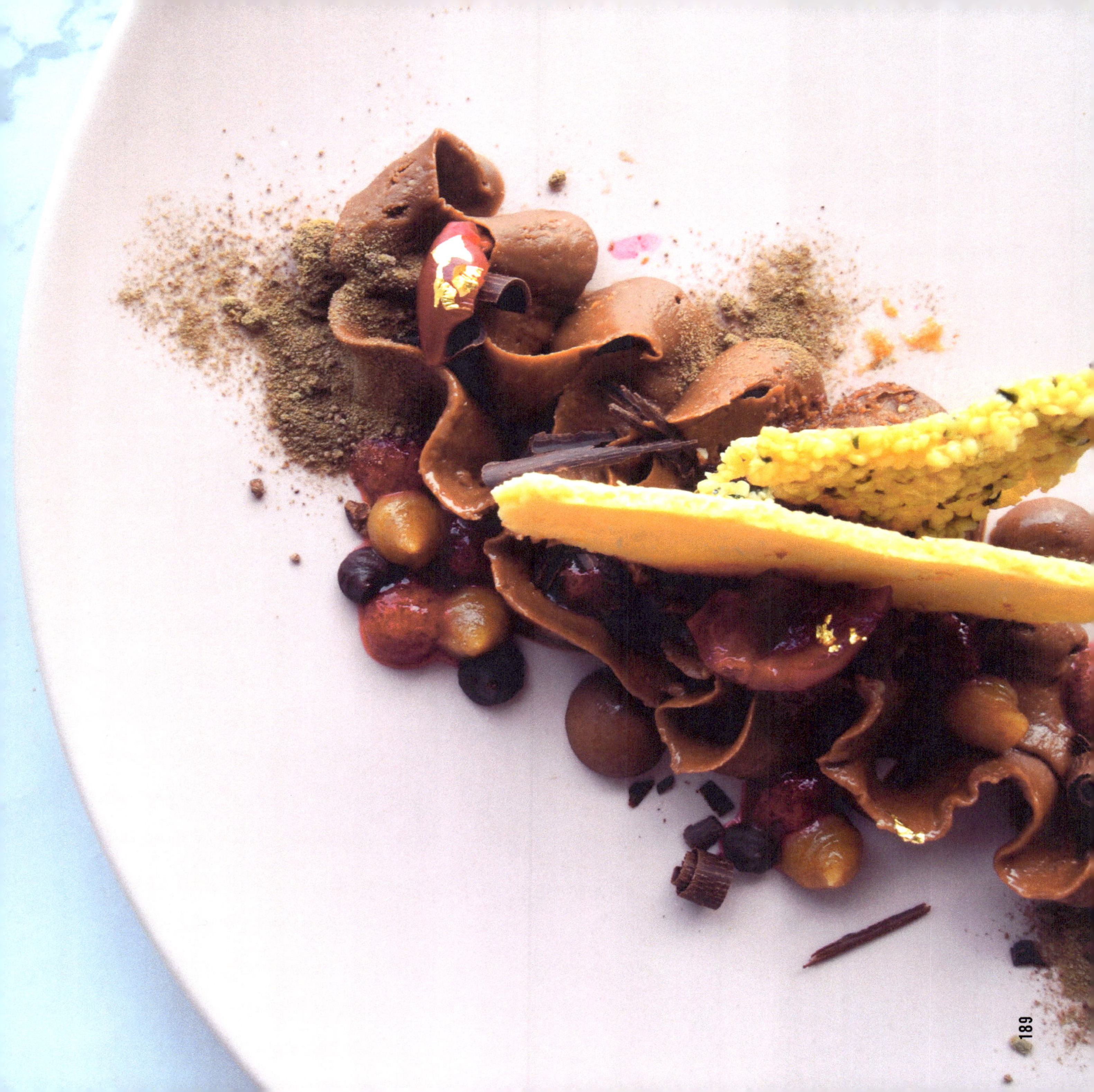

gianduiotto ribbon continued

Instructions

To make gianduiotto

1. Melt the raw chocolate over the bain marie, check the temperature with an infrared thermometer and keep it around 40-42° C. Once melted set aside for 3-4 minutes to cool enough to work with.
2. Place unroasted hazelnut butter to your Blendtec twister or a high speed blender.
3. Add the melted chocolate into the hazelnut butter.
4. Blend well until smooth.
5. Transfer mixture to a pipping bag with Ateco 150 ribbon pastry tube. If it it too fluid, let it sit in the fridge for 5-10 minutes or until becomes easy to pipe.

To make hemp snap

1. Place hemp hearts and light agave into a bowl. Mix well until combined well.
2. Spread mixture onto the dehydrator sheet lined silicon paper.
3. Dehydrate for 8-10 hours at 42° C or until completely crispy.

To make cherry fluid gel

1. Place cherries to your blender. Blend until puree.
2. Add the agave and psyllium husk and blend well.
3. Transfer to a bowl. Let it sit in the fridge for 15-20 minutes until psyllium absorbs the water and the gel becomes thick.
4. Once ready to use, transfer to a pipping bag and set aside.

To make salted caramel

1. In a high speed blender, combine the soaked and drained medjool dates, nut butter, plant milk and salt until smooth and creamy, scraping down the sides of the blender as needed.
2. Transfer mixture in a pipping bag, keep in the refrigerator for 5-10 minutes to set the consistency for pipping.

To make meringue shard

1. Place soaked and drained macadamias to a high speed blender preferably Blendtec twister jar.
2. Add the rest of the ingredients except cacao butter. Blend well until smooth.
3. Melt the cacao butter over bain marie. Then transfer into the mixture. Blend until well combined.
4. Spread mixture onto the dehydrator tray lined silicon sheet. Dehydrate at 42° C for 18-20 hours or until completely dried.
5. Once done, place them into an airtight container and keep in the refrigerator overnight. This process makes them very crispy and delicious.

To make black chocolate soil

1. Grind the chocolate and coconut sugar in a coffee grinder.
2. Transfer to a small food processor, add the charcoal powder. Blend until combined.
3. Keep the soil in a clean and dry jar.

Assembly

1. Once gianduiotto is ready to pipe, pipe it onto the plate in ribbon shape.
2. Place halved cherries around the ribbon.
3. Pipe cherry fluid in dots around the ribbon. You don't need to use any type of pipping tip for the caramel and cherry dots. Just make a small cut to the pipping bag.
4. Pipe salted caramel next to the cherry dots.
5. Cut the meringue shard and hemp snap, place to the next ribbon.
6. Add 1 tbsp black chocolate soil.
7. Using a peeler, shave the chocolate, put some on the ribbon.
8. Using a chef tweezer, decorate with edible gold leaf.
9. Serve immediately!

PS: Check the next page to see different presentation of the same dessert and get some inspiration. We have used whirlpool silicon mould for the gianduiotto, broken into pieces and perfectly paired with same elements in the recipe.

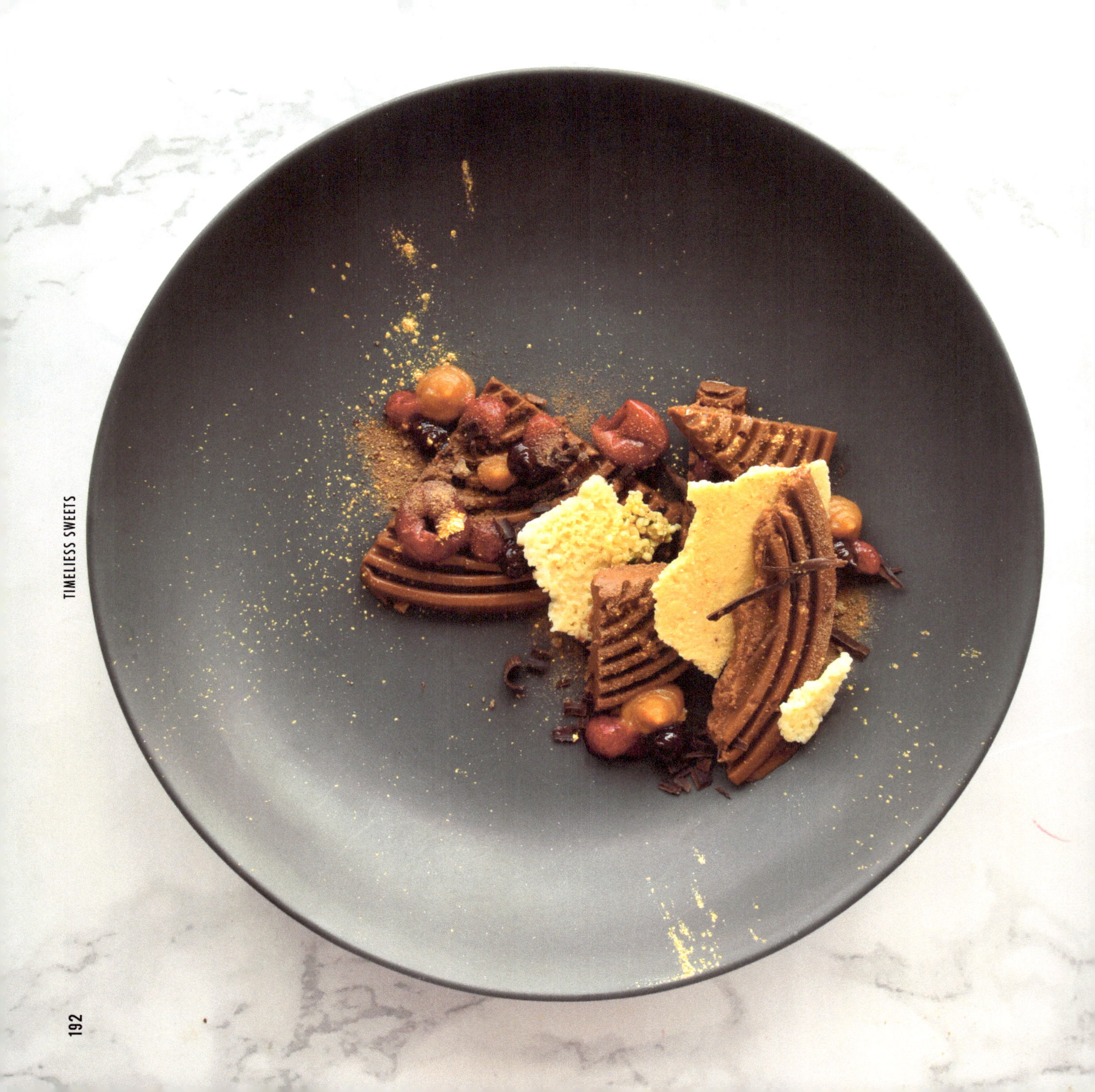

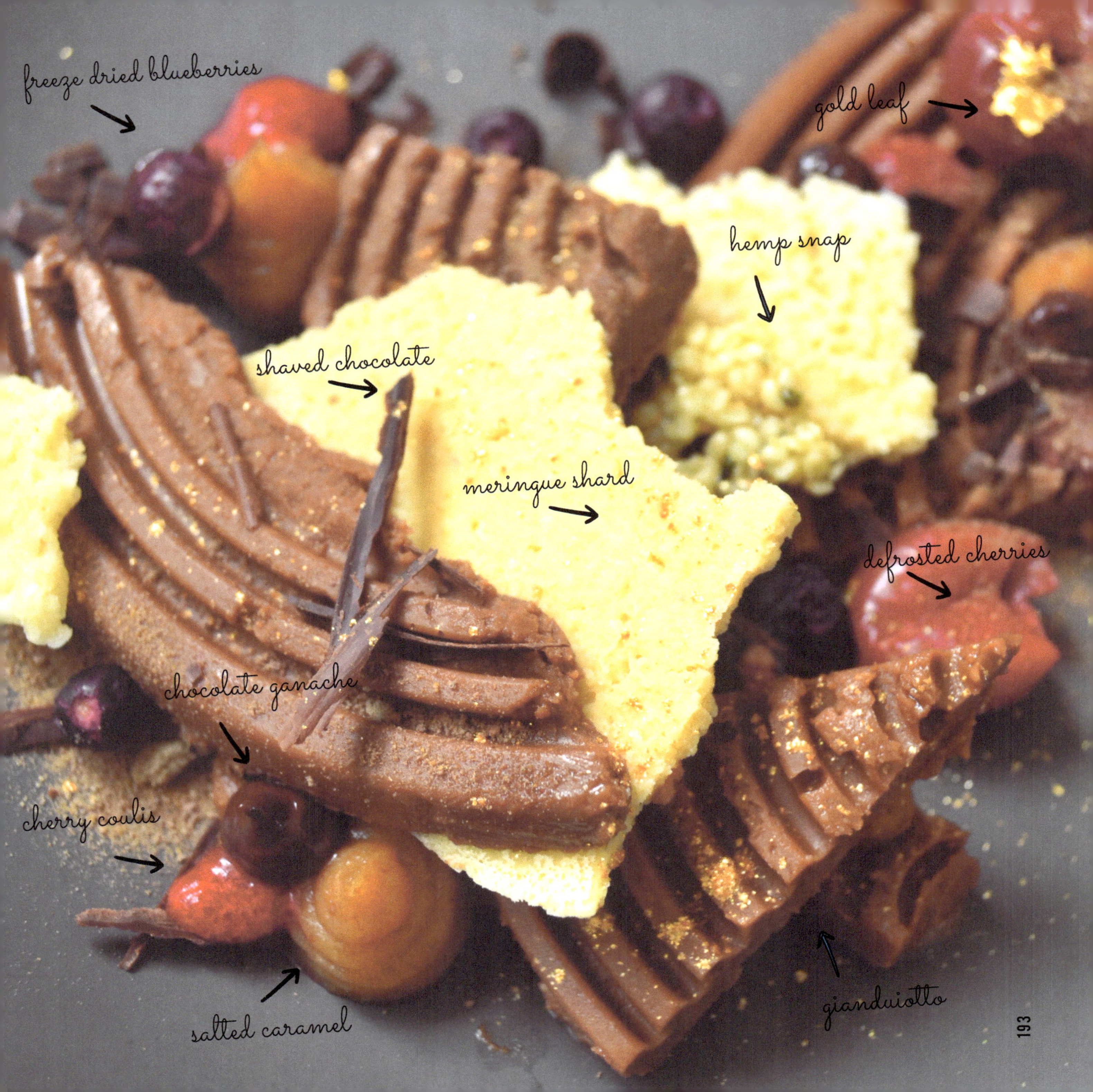
freeze dried blueberries
gold leaf
hemp snap
shaved chocolate
meringue shard
defrosted cherries
chocolate ganache
cherry coulis
salted caramel
gianduiotto

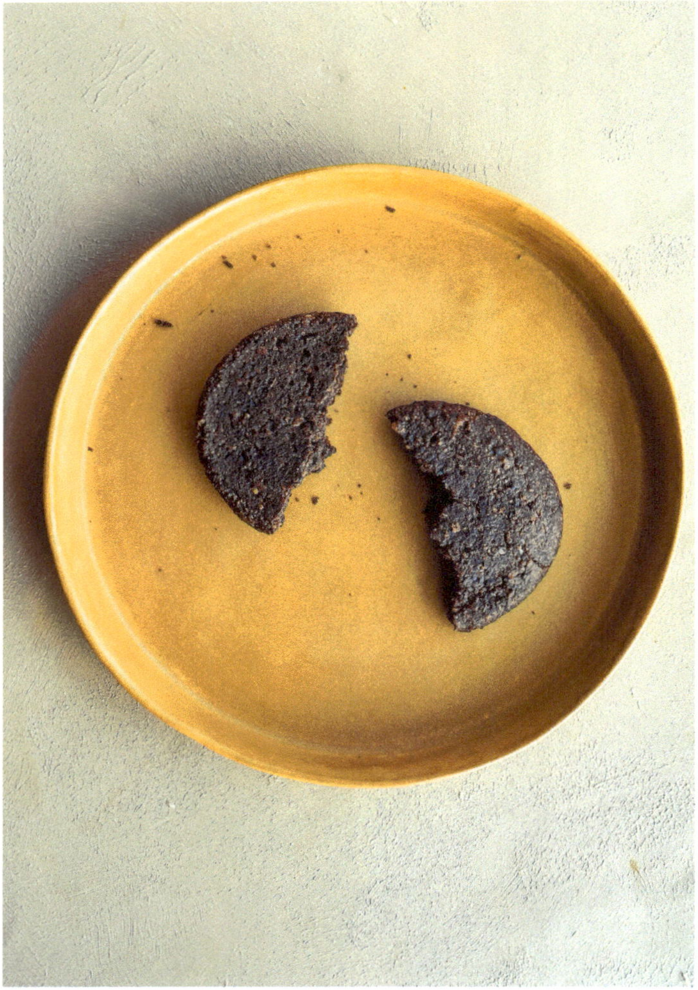

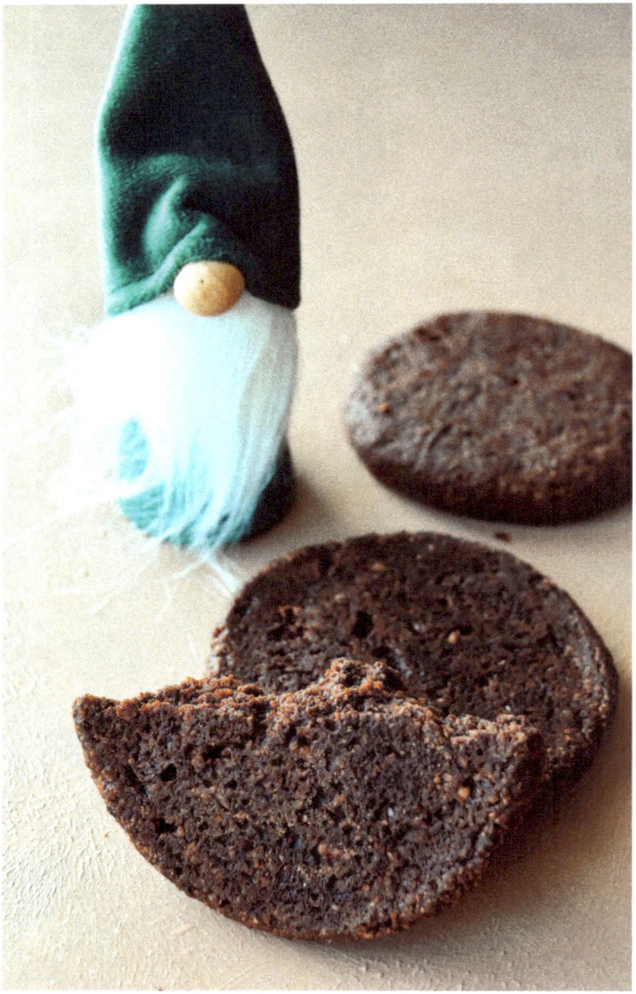

CHOCOLATE COOKIES

Category - Dehydrated-Raw
Time - 10 min prep + 10 hrs dehydration
Quantity - 6 cm 4 pieces

Equipment - Dehydrator
Personal note - The best raw cookies similar to regular ones.

Ingredients

1 tsp chia seeds + 2 tbsp water
1/2 cup sprouted oat flour
2 tbsp raw cacao
1/2 tbsp raw coconut sugar
2 tbsp maple syrup
2 tbsp unroasted hazelnut butter
1 tsp extra virgin olive oil
1/4 tsp salt
1/4 tsp baking soda
40 g finely chopped raw chocolate

Instructions

1. In a mixing bowl, mix chia seeds and water. Keep stirring for the first minute or so to prevent the chia seeds from clumping together. Then set asid for 5 minutes.
3. Then add the rest of ingredients in the chia seed mixture. Stir well to combine.
4. Fold in the chopped raw chocolate.
5. Transfer the dough onto a baking tray lined parchment paper. Lightly wet your hands with a little bit olive oil and shape the dough into small cookies. (6cm X 4 pieces) The cookie won't spread, so shape it the way you want the end result to look like.
6. Dehydrate for 8-10 hours (or overnight) until fully dried both sides of the cookies in the Excalibur dehydrator.
7. It can be stored in the airtight container or jar up to 2 months. Once opened the jar, consume immediately for the best taste.

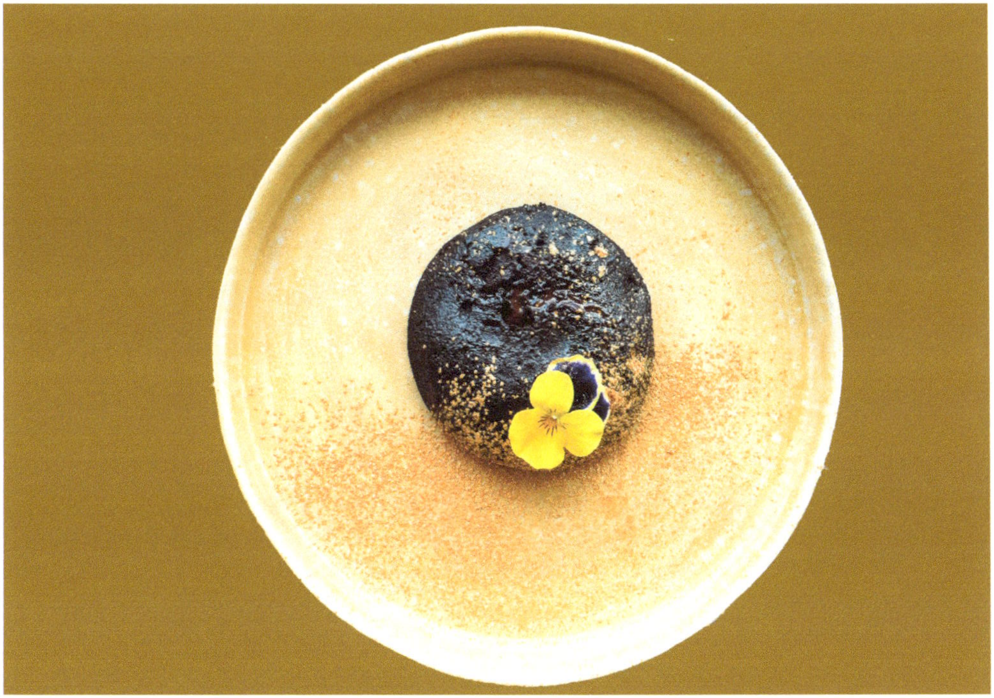

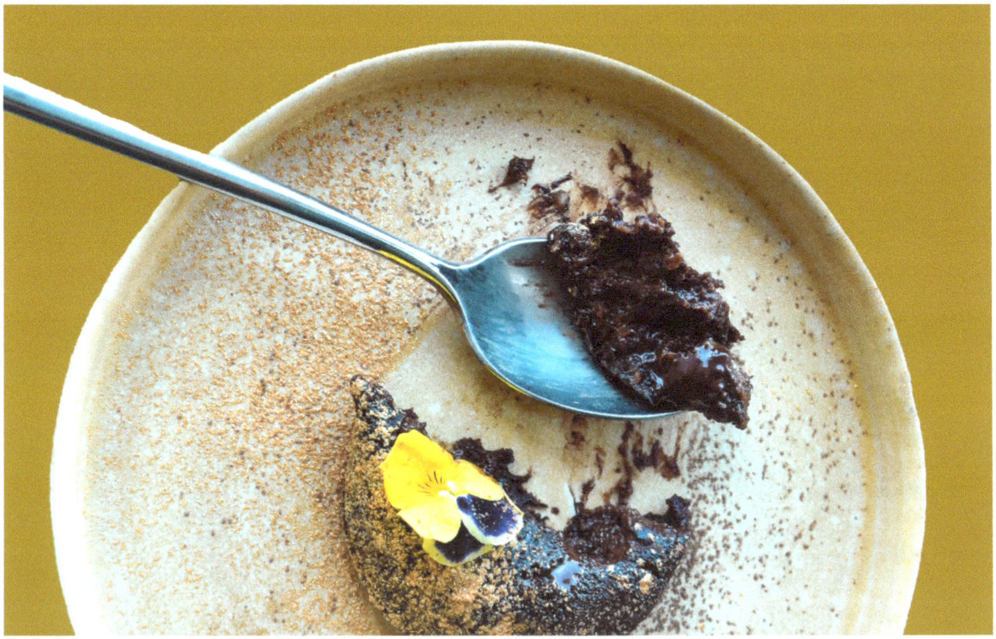

CHOCOLATE FONDANT

Category - Dehydrated-Raw
Time - 10 min prep + 10 hrs dehydration
Quantity - 6 cm 4 pieces

Equipment - Dehydrator, 3 inches x 2 soufflé molds
Personal note - A whole new satisfying experience of eating raw!

Dry Ingredients
50 g cup oat flour
40 g coconut sugar
15 g raw cacao powder
1/2 tsp baking soda

Wet Ingredients
60 g banana
80 g almond milk
25 g almond butter
1/2 tsp apple cider vinegar

Garnish
Raw cacao
Edible gold powder and flowers

Filling
50 g raw chocolate

Instructions
1. Lightly grease 2 small soufflé mold (3 inches in diameter) with olive oil.
2. Mix the dry ingredients in a bowl.
3. In another bowl, mash the banana with a fork. Then add the almond butter.
4. Add the almond milk and apple cider vinegar then mix well.
5. Add the wet to the dry ingredients and combine together.
6. Pour some half of the batter into each soufflé mold.
7. Add the almond butter and a piece of chocolate on top.
8. Cover with the rest of the batter.
9. In dehydrator at 46 C, bake for 6-7 hours. Once baked, remove the mold by inverting it onto the plate.
10. Using bain marie method, melt the raw chocolate, transfer to a piping bag or syringe. Pour the melted raw chocolate inside of the chocolate fondant from the top.
11. Dust some raw cacao and edible gold powder on top. Serve immediately!

index

acknowledgments

Thank you to everyone all over the world who purchased our cookbooks last year and our sponsors who allowed us discover their unique products, we are so grateful for your love and support.

This book "MAD ABOUT RAW" is about spreading the LOVE - not romantic love, not possessive love, not a love of objects or anything outside of ourselves. It is about the love that is everywhere, all the time, within; it is about connecting with mother earth and connecting with each other. We believe you will feel this love much deeper on a raw food diet as it triggers a transformative process that allows you to rebuild yourself at a deep level. Raw plant foods, laughter, joy, gratitude, bliss and unconditional love all exist on the same frequency and make us more grounded and connected to the earth and our higher self. Thank you for purchasing this book and helping us with our mission and our message. We are so blessed to still be making books today!

Much love!

about the author

Nazlı Develi is a food designer, an inventive, aesthetically minded hands-on chef and artist with an eye for details and the creator behind the gurmevegan.com and the founder of GREEN & AWAKE Plant Food Design Studio - greenandawake.com

She specialized in raw vegan cuisine, restaurant consultancy, food design, recipe development, tasting events, workshops, chef training and creative concepts, all rooted in food expression with nature as a core.

Obsessed with art, design, health, wellness and experimental flavours, she's strongly committed to spreading awareness about plant-based food as the most sustainable and necessary alternative for the planet!

Follow on instagram: @gurmevegan I @greenandawake

CPSIA information can be obtained
at www.ICGtesting.com
Printed in the USA
BVHW020118270822
645588BV00008B/831

* 9 7 8 1 7 3 6 3 7 4 2 8 3 *